Control High Blood Pressure Without Drugs

A COMPLETE HYPERTENSION HANDBOOK

Revised and Updated

Robert L. Rowan, M.D.,
with Constance Schrader

A FIRESIDE BOOK

PUBLISHED BY SIMON & SCHUSTER

New York · London · Toronto · Sydney · Singapore

To Agnes Birnbaum of Bleecker Street Associates

for her efforts on behalf of her authors

 FIRESIDE
Rockefeller Center
1230 Avenue of the Americas
New York, NY 10020

FIRESIDE and colophon are registered trademarks
of Simon & Schuster, Inc.

DESIGNED BY JILL WEBER

Manufactured in the United States of America

10 9 8 7 6 5

Library of Congress Cataloging-in-Publication Data

Rowan, Robert L.
  Control high blood pressure without drugs : a complete
hypertension handbook / Robert L. Rowan, with
Constance Schrader.—Revised and updated.
    p.   cm.
    1. Hypertension—Popular works.   2. Hypertension—
Alternative treatment.   I. Schrader, Constance, 1933–
II. Title.

RC685.H8 R69 2001
616.1'3206—dc21   2001023068
ISBN 0-684-87328-1

This book is not intended as a substitute for the medical advice of physicians. The reader should regularly consult a physician in matters relating to his/her health and particularly with respect to any symptoms that may require diagnosis or medical attention.

CONTENTS

$\mathscr{P}$REFACE

This book is the result of fifty years of medical practice, during which I've treated hundreds of patients and conferred with dozens of other physicians, attended conferences, and reviewed medical journals, papers, and other research. It is also the result of my efforts to communicate better with my patients who come to me seeking better health.

It all started half a century ago. I graduated from the University of Virginia School of Medicine in 1950. During these past five decades I've witnessed the wonderful advances in our understanding of how the human body works and in every aspect of medicine and patient care. Years ago, we had very few methods of seeing within the body without invasive surgery. Some tests, such as those for glaucoma, as well as mammography and magnetic or sound imaging, were unavailable and some were unimaginable. Many medicines we have at our disposal now were unheard of at that time. Even the practice of medicine was different in some ways. However, some things have not changed at all: The close and trusting relationship between doctor and patient has always been the same; it is the crux of medical art.

Until recently, preventing disease received little attention. But times have changed. Improving your diet, exercising, and getting regular checkups are now an individual's responsibility. People with chronic diseases, like high blood pressure, can prevent further disability, and in some cases, control the progress of the disease.

I have been fortunate because I have been able to see these advances in medicine, and to use these developing strategies and theories to improve the quality of life for my patients. It has been a blessing to have had the opportunity to help other human beings.

My intense interest in hypertension was inspired by the two years I spent as a drug monitor for Schering Corporation during their development of an antihypertensive drug. This experience increased my respect for scientists and researchers who toil long and hard to create effective and useful medicines. The fact that this book is devoted to the nondrug treatment of hypertension in no way diminishes my belief in the value of medication in many situations. But there are many nondrug activities you can—and should—do for yourself.

My goal in this self-help book is to review accepted practice and to present to you the most recent and reliable medical information. It is a book of real strategies for busy and hurried people who must cope with real-life situations.

Strategies for weight reduction, incorporating exercise into your life, and stress management are presented in the context of today's lifestyles. The beeper you wear on your belt, or the telephone that rings in your pocket are samples of the most recent stressors applied to your body. Appealing new foods are introduced in supermarkets and restaurants almost every month, but which are right for you and your body? A careful selection of foods and beverages is important. I've tried to guide you to the answer.

Perhaps one of the greatest changes has been the acceptance of alternative medicine. About a dozen years ago I wrote about a new concept known as biofeedback. Today it is a well-known and well-accepted technique. Other ideas, some from other cultures, such as acupuncture, and some ancient but newly popular, such as the use of herbal supplements, have been added to the arsenal of weapons we use against disease. In fact, 40 percent of all Americans today use some type of alternative medical therapy along with standard traditional care.

All these advances are exciting and open many options in treatment. It makes me think back on the teachers and colleagues who have been supportive throughout the years. Many physicians have contributed to my education and experience through the years: I will always be indebted to Dean Harvey E. Jordan, Ph.D., who accepted me into medical school; Dr. Thomas Howley, who appointed me to the staff of St. Vincent's Hospital of New York City; and Dr. Pablo Morales, who invited me to teach at the New York University Medical School. I am particularly proud of the time I spent in the U.S. Navy during the Korean War because it allowed me, in a small way, to repay the country that has done so much for me.

I thank my agent, Agnes Birnbaum, who is a tireless advocate for the reader as well as the author and publisher. Through Ms. Birnbaum I met Constance Schrader, who has helped me put my ideas and advice into written words. We hope this book will be your best medicine for controlling high blood pressure.

—ROBERT L. ROWAN, M.D.
New York City, March 2001

PART I

The Basics

The facts behind the disease called hypertension are here. Many of those who suffer from hypertension are unaware that they have it. But once you know you have this disease, you can fight it, and add many years to your life.

CHAPTER 1

Could You Have Hypertension?

Millions of Americans—about one in every four adults, as many as 50 million people—have high blood pressure (HBP). The medical name for high blood pressure is hypertension.

High blood pressure is serious. Hypertension increases the risk of becoming a victim of several life-threatening diseases, including heart and kidney disease and stroke. Having HBP also increases the severity of other diseases and diminishes the general quality of life. Hypertension is especially dangerous because it often gives no warning signs or symptoms.

Do you, or does anyone in your family, have high blood pressure? Many people do have HBP but don't know it until a major illness, such as a heart attack or a stroke, occurs. Unfortunately, hypertension will not "just go away." Fortunately, however, this silent killer *does* respond to management. You *can* do something about hypertension.

Knowledge Is Power (Over Blood Pressure)

Because hypertension is so often a symptomless disorder, the only sure way to tell if you have this disease is to have your blood pressure taken, and to discuss the blood pressure reading with your doctor. Even if your results are in the normal range, you should have your blood pressure checked at least every year. Some simple steps can lower your blood pressure (BP) and can keep your pressure from becoming high if it is normal now.

Only 20 percent of American adults with high blood pressure have it under control. Knowing how your body works will give you the power to prolong your life expectancy and enhance the quality of your life.

What Does "High Blood Pressure" Mean?

Your heart pumps blood to all of your body's organs and tissues, including your brain, in hoselike vessels called arteries. Each time your heart beats— about 60 to 70 times a minute when you are relaxed or resting—it pumps 3 to 4 ounces of blood into your arteries. Blood pressure is the force (pressure) of the blood pushing against the walls of your arteries. Hypertension is a condition in which the pressure of the blood in the arteries exceeds the pressure that is normal and tolerable for your body.

The volume of blood pumped by the heart adds up over the years. Your heart, when you are at rest, pushes about:

1½ gallons of blood through your circulatory system every minute

87 gallons every hour

2,100 gallons every day

766,00 gallons in a year

Millions of gallons during your lifetime

Here is another way of thinking about the blood that pulses through your body: The amount of blood the heart pumps in an average lifetime could fill an artery with the diameter of a drinking straw 300,000 miles long, or about twelve times around the earth at the equator.

Several years ago, a group of volunteers were fitted with a device to record their blood pressure at five-minute intervals during their regular daily routines. Depending on what they were doing their blood pressures showed wide swings up and down. Sitting, sleeping, playing with their pets, and some kinds of mental work made their pressure drop. Driving a car, sexual intercourse, and stressful frustration made their pressure rise. Interestingly, the researchers noted that at some point during the experiment, everyone—even those with normal blood pressure overall—had what could be considered high blood pressure. For instance, during sexual intercourse, the heart rate increases and the blood pressure jumps about 50 percent.

The Symptoms of High Blood Pressure Are Subtle

Most often, there are no symptoms to warn of hypertension. Many people with high blood pressure feel every bit as well as those whose pressure is normal. But certain subtle signs should not be ignored:

Nosebleeds

Dizziness

Ringing in the ears

Fainting spells

Morning headache

Blurred vision

Depression

Urinating at night

Any one of these symptoms can indicate high blood pressure. Because these physical symptoms are so common, it is hard to tie them directly with hypertension. But these symptoms should lead people to consult their doctors, who can then determine whether the patient has hypertension during the medical checkup.

Complaints such as nosebleeds are commonly found in people in the early stages of high blood pressure, unlike the far more serious symptoms of the disease in its later stages, when the body has been damaged. High blood pressure is often the cause of the symptoms listed above. I've seen too many patients with these complaints who turn out to have high blood pressure, and I do not believe their presence together is coincidental. Readers: Please seek medical attention if you have any of these symptoms.

You are your own first line of defense in the battle for your health. If you get nothing else from this book but the stimulus to have your blood pressure checked regularly, you will have received more than your money's worth, and perhaps added years of vigor and health to your life.

Understanding High Blood Pressure

To understand how hypertension occurs, picture a garden hose attached to a faucet, through which water flows, watering the lawn. Now place your foot on the hose near its far end, slowly applying pressure and cutting down the flow of water within the hose. As you increase the pressure with your foot, the pressure of the water within the hose starts to rise. Eventually the pressure will cause the hose to rupture, especially if there is a weak area within its walls. This is essentially what happens when the arterioles (the smallest arteries) begin to block the flow of blood.

When the blood vessel walls face continual high pressure, they thicken. We do not yet understand how this comes about. It may result from an increase in the number of muscle cells that compose the wall, or from an increase of fluid within the cells. Many experts think that thickening of the arterial wall follows a kidney malfunction, which increases the amount of water retained in the body.

Who Is Most at Risk?

Here are some of the factors that raise your risk of having or developing high blood pressure:

Age: Anyone can have hypertension, but older people are most susceptible. Among Americans age sixty-five or older, more than half have high blood pressure. Although age plays an important role in this disease, hypertension can develop in people younger than twenty. Normal pressure readings in children are not usually as high as readings found in adults; young people are considered to have hypertension when their blood pressure exceeds the normal level for their particular age group. Under the age of fifty, hypertension is more common in men than in women. After fifty-five or sixty, it is more likely to strike females than males. However, women tolerate high blood pressure better than men, and more men than women die of high blood pressure.

Genes: African-Americans of every age group have a greater incidence of high blood pressure than white or Hispanic people, according to a U.S. Public Health Service study on health and nutrition. This government organization studied 17,796 people, and found the following incidence of hypertension among whites and blacks:

White men: 18.5 per 100 people

White women: 15.7 per 100 people

Black men: 27.8 per 100 people

Black women: 28.6 per 100 people

Family history: Hypertension often appears in families. If one parent has hypertension, there is a better than average chance their children will also have it; if both parents suffer from the disease, the odds are even higher. Conversely, some people seem to inherit an ability to ward off hypertension. Even with the advances in genetic research, we don't know how heredity accounts for this seeming immunity. In addition, we assume that environment also plays a part. You can inherit a predisposition to develop hypertension but you may need other particular factors to trigger it.

Weight: People who are more than 25 to 30 percent over their ideal body weight are more likely than people who are not overweight to have high normal to mild high blood pressure. Studies have shown that obese people (those whose weight is 30 percent or more above their ideal body weight) are even more likely to develop high blood pressure.

Inactivity: Being a couch potato is not just a joke; it can be detrimental to your health. A sedentary lifestyle contributes to your being overweight. Regular exercise helps in weight control and also relieves stress and anxiety.

Stress: Some people react to stress with a temporary rise in blood pressure. Whether stress can cause chronic hypertension, though, is not completely proven, but many physicians do suspect that stress plays a role in many such cases of high blood pressure. High levels of stress over a long period of time may boost pressure by activating your involuntary nervous system.

Alcohol consumption: Studies have shown that heavy consumption of alcohol can increase blood pressure dramatically.

Smoking: All the evidence indicates smokers are at increased risk for high blood pressure.

Sodium sensitivity: A diet high in salt can accelerate hypertension as we age. Slightly fewer than half of the people with HBP are salt-sensitive, in that they are vulnerable to the effects of sodium on blood pressure. Americans consume far more sodium than their bodies need. When placed on a low-salt diet, many people notice that their blood pressure drops; high-salt diets can also be harmful for people who have low levels of renin, a kidney enzyme that prevents reduction of blood pressure.

At a recent medical symposium sponsored by the National Kidney Foundation, the U.S. Department of Health and Human Services, and the International Life Sciences Institute (an industry group), some experts

Lifestyle a Focus of HBP Study

During January 2000, a *New York Times* article stated that Northern European and American men with high blood pressure are three times more likely to die of a heart attack than men with the same blood pressure from Japan or from the Mediterranean coast of Europe. The news came from a study published in *The New England Journal of Medicine*. This study provides evidence that lifestyle should be the main focus of efforts to lower blood pressure. "If you eliminate the factors that we know about, which are largely lifestyle issues—smoking, high blood pressure, high cholesterol, lack of exercise, and diabetes—you can eliminate somewhere between 70 and 90 percent of disease in our population," states Dr. Richard Pasternak, director of preventive cardiology at Massachusetts General Hospital. He adds, "For a long time, doctors have defined high blood pressure as 140/90 and higher. However, the study adds to a growing body of evidence that people who fall below that mark can benefit significantly by cutting their blood pressure further."

challenged the idea that reducing salt in a normal person's diet reduces the risk for HBP. However, it was agreed that large amounts of sodium in the diets of people predisposed to the disease are harmful. You might best describe the problem by saying, "Some people have a strong sensitivity to salt, and when they eat too much of it, they become hypertensive."

Geography: Where you live makes a difference, although researchers don't know why. High blood pressure is less common in tropical climates, perhaps owing to a relaxed lifestyle. The southeastern states of our country have some of the highest rates of death from stroke, a hypertension-related disease. These eleven states—Alabama, Arkansas, Georgia, Indiana, Kentucky, Louisiana, Mississippi, North Carolina, South Carolina, Tennessee, and Virginia—have such high rates of stroke among people of all ages and racial groups, as well as both sexes, that they are called the "Stroke Belt States."

Other factors: Some researchers believe height makes a difference; the taller a person is, the more pressure might be needed to pump blood, against the pull of gravity, to the brain. Body shape has also been linked to high blood pressure. Sleep apnea, a severe form of snoring that interrupts breathing during sleep, can stress the heart muscle and increase the snorer's hypertension risk. Even a fondness for licorice, which causes the body to retain fluids, can adversely affect your health.

Risk factors—physical conditions and traits or lifestyle habits that significantly correlate with specific diseases—mount up very fast. If you have more than one of these factors, work on the ones you can change. Since you can't change your heredity, try to eliminate any of the factors you can. I have often advised my patients that the best way of treating a disease is to prevent it. Lowering your weight, being as active as possible, quitting smoking, and limiting your drinking are all good ways of lowering your hypertension risk.

Primary (Essential) High Blood Pressure—and Salt

For about 90 percent of the people with hypertension, no single cause of high blood pressure is known. This type of high blood pressure is called primary or essential hypertension. This type of blood pressure can't be cured, although in most cases it can be controlled.

Secondary Hypertension

A few people trace their high blood pressure to a known cause, such as tumors of the adrenal gland, kidney disease, or a hormonal abnormality. This is called secondary hypertension, and it can usually be cured if the trigger can be corrected or passes.

Malignant Hypertension

Especially dangerous is malignant hypertension, where readings can exceed 200/130 mm Hg (these readings are explained fully in Chapter 3). Often this condition is discovered completely by accident, because it usually causes no symptoms or discomfort. (About half the people found to have HBP say they didn't know it.)

Malignant hypertension is so severe that a doctor can sometimes detect it by simply looking into the patient's eyes, since in some cases the optic nerve can hemorrhage and swell. Malignant hypertension can also cause kidney damage, brain swelling, and impaired vision.

Before antihypertensive drugs were developed in the 1950s, many people who developed this deadly form of the disease would die within a year of diagnosis. These days, however, high blood pressure is usually treated well before that stage, and malignant hypertension is seen less often. When it is discovered, there are many new drugs that can treat it.

Hypotension, the Other Side of the Coin

Sometimes blood pressure is below normal. This condition, the opposite of hypertension, is called hypotension. It commonly affects people in shock, although healthy, normal people can suffer its symptoms. Hypotension also signals that you should have your physician check any of your medications. Doctors generally agree that people with low blood pressure have a longer life expectancy than others, since there is less wear and tear on the arteries and heart.

Some very serious effects can result from a decrease in blood pressure due to loss of blood and the development of shock. (Shock can be caused by factors other than the loss of blood.) One condition caused by hypotension that affects the brain results from the G force that occurs when an airplane makes a very sharp turn at a very high speed. The blood of those aboard is pushed out of the head and into the lower part of the body. When this happens, the pilot and the passengers will lose consciousness. It is avoided by the pilot's wearing a G force suit. This garment applies pressure to the lower half of the body, preventing the blood in the head from leaving too quickly, and keeping the blood in balance throughout the body.

In the case of orthostatic hypotension, the brain is deprived of blood as a result of suddenly sitting up or standing after being in a prone position. This causes a sudden but temporary loss of blood to the brain, resulting in a momentary dizziness or loss of consciousness. This situation corrects itself without medical intervention.

Orthostatic hypotension occurs because we do not have stop valves in the blood vessels that feed blood to the brain. Are some animals better suited to fast head movements than we are? Yes. Take the case of the giraffe. Giraffes lower their head about fourteen feet to drink from a stream or water hole. When the sight or smell of a predator alerts the giraffe, he raises his head very suddenly. The giraffe has valves in the blood vessels of his neck that prevent the blood in his head and neck from leaving his brain. We humans were shortchanged in this regard. We should have been given valves in our neck vessels.

Many people with low blood pressure show no symptoms at all. Not all physicians agree that such symptoms as fatigue, dizziness, occasional light-headedness, and blurred vision are caused by hypotension. If you do have any of these symptoms, though, you should have your blood pressure checked.

A good first step in maintaining a healthy life is getting your blood pressure checked on a regular basis. There is no other way to know for sure whether you have this potentially deadly disease called high blood pressure. If you do, this book will guide you, step by step, through what you can do to lessen HBP's harmful effects.

CHAPTER 2

The Dangers of High Blood Pressure

Medical research and statistical charts indicate that if you have high blood pressure, you have increased chances of dying at an earlier age than someone your age without the disease. Although high blood pressure raises your risk of dying too soon, managing your blood pressure has been shown to add years to your life. There is something—in fact there are many things—you can do.

What Are the Dangers of This Silent Killer?

Why do the statistics report such bad news? What's so bad about hypertension? Untreated, hypertension can lead to a frightening list of life-threatening disorders:

ATHEROSCLEROSIS, OR "HARDENING OF THE ARTERIES"

Atherosclerosis is an ongoing disease. The inner walls of the arteries become thick and irregular from deposits of a fatty substance called cholesterol (more on cholesterol in Chapter 12). This thickening of artery walls happens gradually over time, restricting blood flow to vital organs. Some thickening of the artery walls is a natural part of aging, but this effect of the aging process may be slowed through diet and exercise.

Over time, like an old garden hose, arteries can stiffen. It has been difficult to measure this stiffness, but new tests are being developed to gauge it by measuring the speed of pulse waves—the waves of pressure that travel down the artery walls as blood circulates. A computer program translates the timing of the waves into numerical values.

Both atherosclerosis and stiffness of blood vessels increase with age. Is there a link? Normally smooth vascular muscle cells in the artery are constantly contracting and relaxing, giving tone to artery walls. One theory is that stiffness of the blood vessels triggers the process that leads to atherosclerosis.

HEART FAILURE

When the heart is unable to pump the amount of blood needed by the body, heart failure can result. High blood pressure can cause heart failure, which in turn can lead to congestion in the body tissues, with fluid accumulating in the legs, abdomen, and lungs. This condition may develop over a period of years.

ANGINA PECTORIS

Angina, also called angina pectoris, is a chest pain or a sensation of pressure in the chest. It indicates that the heart muscle isn't receiving enough oxygen. The harder and faster a heart works, the more oxygen it needs. When your arteries are narrowed or blocked so that the blood flow cannot meet your heart's needs, you may feel pain in the heart muscle, chest, arm, upper body, or face area.

ACUTE MYOCARDIAL INFARCTION (HEART ATTACK)

The medical term for a heart attack is acute myocardial infarction, medically abbreviated as MI. Heart attack is America's most prevalent killer. A portion of the heart muscle can die when an obstructed coronary artery prevents an adequate oxygen supply from reaching the heart.

ANEURYSM OF THE MAIN BODY ARTERY (THE AORTA)

An aneurysm is a localized abnormal dilation of a blood vessel. The aorta, the largest artery in the body, conducts blood away from the heart, then branches into many smaller arteries throughout the body. With age, the aorta enlarges and its walls become stiffer. An aneurysm can occur in an artery as well.

CEREBROVASCULAR ACCIDENT (STROKE)

High blood pressure is the main cause of stroke. A stroke is a sudden disruption in the flow of blood to an area of the brain. Deprived of blood, the affected brain cells either become damaged or die. While cell damage can often be repaired and the loss of function regained, the death of brain cells is permanent and results in disability. There are three major types of stroke:

The thrombotic stroke is most common. Fatty deposits (plaque) build up in the arteries (blood vessels) that supply blood to the brain. This severely reduces the blood flow until, eventually, a clot or clump (called a thrombus) in an artery entirely blocks the path of blood.

An embolic stroke results when a blood clot forms somewhere else in the body (usually in arteries of the heart or neck), and the clot travels through the circulatory system to the brain. The traveling clot is an embolus.

A hemorrhagic stroke is the most severe type of stroke. It occurs when a blood vessel in the brain bursts, allowing blood to pour into the brain outside normal channels.

KIDNEY FAILURE

As blood flows through your vascular system, it presses against the walls of the blood vessels. Extra fluid in your body increases the volume of fluid in the blood and makes the blood pressure higher. (Narrow or clogged blood vessels also raise blood pressure.) Decreased blood flow can release renin.

High blood pressure makes the heart work hard and can damage blood vessels throughout the body. If the blood vessels in the kidneys are damaged, they may stop doing their job (removing wastes and extra fluid from the blood) and raise fluid levels even more. Second to diabetes, high blood pressure is the leading cause of kidney failure.

Kidney failure may occur when the kidneys are unable adequately to rid the body of toxins. Kidney failure can have many causes. A rapid failure can be triggered by poisoning, as well as decrease in blood supply. Chronic kidney failure is a slow decline in kidney function, and high blood pressure is one of the causes.

Although these serious diseases have many causes, they have been linked with hypertension. Historically, efforts have focused on the detection, evaluation, and treatment of hypertension. There has been a great deal of progress in all of these areas, but the number of people affected by high blood pressure remains large. The good news is that strategies to lower blood pressure are effective, and the same strategies lower the risks of any of these illnesses.

OTHER POSSIBLE HBP-LINKED HEALTH PROBLEMS

Various other medical problems have also been linked to high blood pressure. It can lead to a thickening of the tiny capillaries in the eyes, which restricts blood flow through the eyes, which can lead to tunnel vision or blindness.

A very small percentage of women who use birth control pills develop hypertension, which is reversible when use of the pills is discontinued. The cause of this hypertension is thought to be linked with the body's endocrine system. The condition can also occur because of a rare type of complication of pregnancy called preeclampsia or eclampsia. Eclampsia is a disease occurring at the end of pregnancy in which the blood pressure can rise to 140/90 mm Hg or often higher (see Chapter 3 for an explanation of blood pressure readings). It can lead to severe internal damage to the mother and at times to the fetus. The cause is not understood, and treatment is extremely difficult.

Hypertension can result from brain tumors, which cause increased blood pressure within the head.

High blood pressure can sometimes be noticed directly after surgery, as with coronary bypass surgery. This type can be relieved.

Illegal (street) drugs such as methamphetamine and cocaine can cause a temporary rise in blood pressure. Continued use can damage the kidneys or other organs and lead to severe hypertension.

A recent Duke University Medical Center study has verified the link between hypertension and memory problems. For the study, a group of people between the ages of 29 and 59 completed tests that involved different aspects of memory. Those who suffered from high blood pressure did not perform as well as others in the test group. When blood pressure remains up, life expectancy goes down.

How Much Do You Know About Your Blood Pressure?

Test your knowledge of high blood pressure by answering the following questions. Answer each true or false. The answers are given below.

1. There is nothing you can do to prevent high blood pressure.　　　　　　T　　　F

2. If either of your parents has high blood pressure, you will probably have high blood pressure.　　　　　　T　　　F

3. Young adults don't get high blood pressure.　　　　　　T　　　F

4. High blood pressure has no symptoms.　　　　　　T　　　F

5. Stress causes high blood pressure.　　　　　　T　　　F

6. High blood pressure is not life-threatening.　　　　　　T　　　F

7. Blood pressure is high when it's at or over 140/90 mm Hg.　　　　　　T　　　F

8. If you're overweight you are two to six times more likely to develop high blood pressure.　　　　　　T　　　F

9. You have to exercise vigorously every day to improve your blood pressure.　　　　　　T　　　F

10. Americans eat two or three times more salt than they need.　　　　　　T　　　F

11. Drinking alcohol lowers blood pressure.　　　　　　T　　　F

12. High blood pressure has no cure.　　　　　　T　　　F

Here are the answers and a short explanation of each answer. There is no passing grade on this quiz. The quiz is just a way of giving you more information about high blood pressure.

1. *False:* High blood pressure can be prevented by doing a number of things, most important among them: keep a healthy weight, be physically active, limit your salt use, drink alcoholic beverages only in moderation.

2. *False:* You are more likely to get high blood pressure if it runs in your family, but that doesn't mean you must get it. Your chance of getting high blood pressure is also greater if you're older or an African-American. But high blood pressure is *not* an inevitable part of aging, and everyone can take steps to prevent the disease.

3. *False:* About 7 million people ages eighteen to thirty-nine are among the 50 million Americans with high blood pressure. Once you have high blood pressure, you have it for the rest of your life. If you take steps early, you may be able to avoid hypertension.

4. *True:* High blood pressure usually has no symptoms. In fact, it is often called the silent killer. You can have high blood pressure and feel fine. That's why it's important to have your blood pressure checked.

5. *False:* Stress does make blood pressure go up. Ups and downs in blood pressure are normal. Run for a bus and your pressure rises, sleep and it drops. Blood pressure becomes dangerous, however, when it's always high. That harms your heart and blood vessels. So what does cause high blood pressure? In the majority of cases, a single cause is never found.

6. *False:* High blood pressure is the main cause of stroke. It is also a factor in the development of heart disease and kidney failure.

7. *True:* But even blood pressure slightly under 140/90 mm Hg can increase your risk of heart disease or stroke. More about the way blood pressure is measured can be found in Chapter 3.

8. *True:* As weight increases, so does blood pressure. It's important to stay at a healthy weight. If you need to reduce, try to lose one half to one pound a week. Choose foods low in fat, especially saturated fat, since fat is high in calories. Even if you're at a good weight, the healthiest way to eat is low-fat, low-cholesterol foods. Calories do count.

9. *False:* Studies show that even a little physical activity helps prevent high blood pressure and strengthens your heart. Even among the overweight, those who are active have lower blood pressure than those who aren't. It's best to do some activity for thirty minutes most days. Walk, garden, or participate in sports. If you don't have a thirty-minute period, fifteen minutes twice a day is a good start. Every bit of activity helps. Make movement and motion part of your daily routine.

10. *True:* Salt is made of sodium and chloride, and it's mostly the sodium that affects blood pressure. Americans eat too much salt. Some people are especially sensitive to sodium. Salt is added to foods at the table and in cooking. Sodium and salt are used in processed food and snacks. People with high blood pressure should eat no more than 6 grams of salt a day, which equals about 2,400 milligrams of sodium.

11. *False:* Drinking alcoholic beverages can raise blood pressure. No more than two drinks a day if you are a man, and one drink a day if you are a woman, if you must. A drink is 1.5 ounces of 80 proof whiskey, 5 ounces of wine, or 12 ounces of beer.

12. *True:* High blood pressure can be treated and controlled. Treatment usually includes basic lifestyle changes, such as losing weight, becoming physically active, limiting salt, stopping smoking, and avoiding drinking more than one alcoholic beverage a day, and, if needed, taking medication that your physician prescribes. But the best way to avoid the dangers of high blood pressure is to prevent the condition in the first place by adopting a healthy lifestyle. Throughout this book you will see that yes, you do have the power to change your lifestyle and improve your health.

CHAPTER 3

Measure Your Pressure

Even with the wonderful advances in medical science, high blood pressure has no cure. Once high blood pressure occurs, it usually continues a lifetime. However, there is good news! You can lower your blood pressure with treatment and with lifestyle changes. But if you stop treatment and/or return to your original lifestyle, it will go up again. If members of your family have high blood pressure, it is best to be vigilant on your and their behalf. Or if you have any of the diseases that have been linked to hypertension, you should be especially careful.

First, find out if your blood pressure is high. Checking your blood pressure is painless and takes only minutes. If you have hypertension the results will be the basis on which to make your plans.

How Is Blood Pressure Measured?

Having your blood pressure checked is quick and easy. Blood pressure is measured with an instrument called a sphygmomanometer (pronounced *sfig*-mo ma-*nom*-e-ter). The word comes from the Greek "sphygmos," meaning pulse, and "metron," meaning measure. A blood pressure cuff is wrapped around your upper arm and inflated to stop the blood flow in your artery for a few seconds. A valve is opened releasing air from the cuff. The sounds of blood rushing through an artery are heard through a stethoscope. The first sound heard and registered on the gauge or mercury column is called the *systolic blood pressure.* This represents the maximum pressure in the artery, produced as the heart contracts and the blood begins to flow. The last sound heard, as more air is released from the cuff, is the *diastolic blood pressure*. This represents the lowest pressure that remains within the artery when the heart is at rest.

When your health care professional tells you what your blood pressure is, he or she might say numbers such as "120 over 80." Hypertension is usually defined as resting blood pressure greater than 140/90, or "140 over 90." However, elderly people often have blood pressure readings above these numbers, and young children often have blood pressure well below these readings.

Your blood pressure is highest when the left ventricle of the heart contracts. At that instant, the heart is said to be in *systole*. The pressure is lowest when the heart is at rest. At that instant, it is said to be in *diastole*. The diastolic pressure is often considered significant because it defines the lowest constant pressure on the arteries.

PRESSURE BY THE NUMBERS

The numbers used in measuring blood pressure refer to the distance, in millimeters (mm), that the pressure within your system would push a column of mercury (Hg) upward. (You may wonder why I talk about millimeters of mercury when you don't see mercury in the instrument used to measure blood pressure. Years ago, mercury was used in sphygmomanometers; today instruments use air pressure equal to that of mercury, although some doctors still use the mercury-style apparatus. Both models are equally dependable.)

When blood pressure is checked at your doctor's office or as part of a health care checkup, you learn something about what is happening within your body. The stethoscope is one of the most used, and most valuable, tools of medical science.

New devices use blood pressure cuffs plus digital readout or electronic devices. Many use microphones or some other sensing devices instead of a stethoscope. All properly calibrated instruments give reasonably accurate blood pressure readings.

THE MEANING OF THE NUMBERS

In hypertension, the force exerted by the blood pressing against the artery wall is above the level considered normal. Until recently, the National Heart, Lung, and Blood Institute, which is part of the National Institutes of Health, considered a pressure of 160/95 to be hypertension and the range between 140/90 and 160/95 to be borderline hypertension. These demarcations are inaccurate, for any sustained rise in pressure can indicate hypertension, and medical monitoring is the best course of action. The latest classifications of hypertension are as follows:

Normal blood pressure: 80 to 89 diastolic pressure

Mild hypertension: 90 to 104 diastolic pressure

Moderate hypertension: 105 to 114 diastolic pressure

Severe hypertension: above 114 diastolic pressure

CLASSIFICATION OF BLOOD PRESSURE FOR ADULTS

SYSTOLIC MM HG (TOP NUMBER)	DIASTOLIC MM HG (BOTTOM NUMBER)	CLASSIFICATION	FOLLOW-UP
130 or lower	84 or lower	normal	recheck every year
130–139	85–89	high normal	recheck every year, begin some lifestyle modification to avoid high blood pressure
140–159	90–99	Stage 1	recheck in two months
160–179	100–109	Stage 2	see doctor
180–209	110–119	Stage 3	see doctor
210 or higher	120 or higher	Stage 4	see doctor immediately

Note: *Use the higher classification when the systolic and diastolic pressures fall into different stages. Elderly people often have blood pressure above these readings, and young children have blood pressure below these readings.*

White Coat Hypertension

Some patients are anxious every time they have their blood pressure measured. They know it is painless, and they assure me they are not afraid, but their blood pressure goes up. This reaction is not unusual. Other physicians have also recognized this reaction.

The question is, does blood pressure increase only when a "white coat" (any health care person who takes the patient's pressure) approaches, or does it happen whenever a tense situation arises? So far, most studies have found the condition to be limited to medical settings. People with white coat hypertension usually respond to other stress factors the same way other people do. Most people with white coat hypertension don't respond with anxiety and higher pressure numbers when they take their own blood pressure, or when they use machines in stores or malls. (Note: Machines may be accurate when they are installed in stores, but they lose accuracy over time, since they tend to be misused and not maintained properly.)

If your doctor suspects your high blood pressure is linked to medical situations, he or she may recommend that you wear a portable device that measures pressure periodically. Or you can learn to take your own blood pressure at home, a low-stress environment.

Monitoring Blood Pressure Yourself

Your blood pressure reading can be taken quickly and accurately outside a clinical setting. In the past few years, many blood pressure monitors have been introduced, and many more are now in development. The devices are getting smaller, more accurate, and easier to use, as well as less expensive. (At present, you can buy a home device for between $20 and $100. Several medical groups are lobbying to make the devices available under Medicare and Medicaid.) Most manufacturers also have smaller or larger than average-sized cuffs available. If your doctor or health care provider has encouraged you to monitor your own blood pressure, you'll need a measuring device. Here are the basic types:

+ The mercury sphygmomanometer is the traditional BP measurement device. It is large, has a long glass gauge, and will give you consistent, accurate readings. Unfortunately, it is big and bulky for home use, and hazardous because of the mercury in the gauge, although some models have an unbreakable tube.

- Aneroid—using no liquid—equipment is inexpensive, portable, and lightweight. Some models have an easy-reading large gauge and a D-cuff that is easy to control. Unfortunately, the mechanism is delicate and must be checked often for accuracy. When damaged, it requires factory repair and readjustment.

- Electronic or digital equipment is contained in one unit, and so requires less dexterity than other devices. Some models have a D-ring cuff for one-handed application or a cuff that fits around the wrist, automatic inflation and deflation systems, and best of all for anyone with hearing problems, an easy-to-read digital display. Some models have printouts and built-in pulse measurements. Some of these devices are extremely sensitive.

- In recent years, a development called fuzzy logic has become very popular in devices for monitoring blood pressure. Fuzzy logic refers to a built-in technology that enables the blood pressure monitor to "think" for the user. You simply push the start button and the monitor makes ongoing adjustments as it inflates until it reaches the ideal cuff inflation for your arm or wrist. Note: Digital blood pressure monitors use a computer to obtain blood pressure readings, rather than monitoring sounds. In the computer method, a computer chip calculates a blood pressure reading based on a wave that it picks up from the cuff.

- Wrist blood pressure monitors are recommended for people with arthritis or other ailments that make an arm model too difficult to use. Wrist monitors are all relatively small and easy to carry. Finger blood pressure monitors are also available, but I usually recommend them only when my patient cannot use the arm or wrist style.

Your local pharmacy may stock some BP monitoring devices, or you can order from a medical supply company. Ask your doctor or pharmacist for help. When you think you have mastered the use of the device, take it to your doctor to check it, and to be sure you are using it and reading it correctly. Remember: Home blood pressure measurement is no substitute for periodic evaluation by your doctor.

KEEPING BP RECORDS

Home blood pressure monitors described above can be a tool in managing your hypertension. They will let you know your blood pressure level and alert you to possible problems. If you use a home monitor, you should record your blood pressure and pulse reading in a notebook daily. When you next visit your physician, it will be a big help in working together to manage your condition and spot any changes.

Don't panic if you have an unusually low or high blood pressure reading. It is important to speak with your physician to learn what range is normal for you and to repeat any measurements that seem abnormal after waiting about ten minutes. Also, by measuring your blood pressure at the same time every day, it will be easier to compare readings.

Measuring Your Own Blood Pressure—The Method

Using a home blood pressure monitor can be an important tool in the management of hypertension as well as hypotension (low blood pressure). Ideally, blood pressure should be taken with the arm bare. A tight sleeve constricts your arm or makes it impossible for the blood pressure cuff to fit properly. If you use a home monitor, follow all the directions on the machine as carefully as possible. Following are some general directions for an arm-band sphygmomanometer.

- You must wrap the cuff around your arm about one inch above the crease in your skin at the elbow. After you have placed this cuff, force air into it by pumping the rubbery bulb attached to it via a tubing. The cuff should be snug, but there should be enough room for you to slip one fingertip under the cuff. If the cuff doesn't fit, the readings will be incorrect. The small round disk you see is an air pressure valve, which you can open and close by simple turning. It will require a few moments of experimentation until you are able to fill the cuff comfortably with air and then release it in a slow, controlled manner.

- Next, you must locate the artery in your forearm from which you will hear the sounds of your blood pressure. This is the brachial artery and is found within the crease of your forearm at the level of the elbow. You can find the brachial artery by extending your left arm in front of you and feeling for an area near your elbow, about two inches from the inside part of your arm. Use the second, third, and fourth fingers of your right hand to find this area.

- You may have to continue to straighten your left arm to its full length to find the brachial artery. The location must be accurate, for you need to place the end of the stethoscope directly over this artery for accurate reading. Do not apply too much pressure or you will close off the artery, defeating the purpose of the stethoscope. Apply only enough pressure to listen to the artery but not to cut off the flow.

♦ Place the earpieces of the stethoscope in both ears. Note that the ends point upward to match your ear canals. If you put the earpieces in upside down, they will not fit comfortably.

♦ Finally, pump the cuff to a level that completely blocks any sound coming from the artery. Now slowly drop the pressure, about 2 to 3 millimeters every few seconds; this will require a little practice. The first sounds you hear will tell you the level of the systolic blood pressure. Keep listening, and keep lowering the pressure; you will find that eventually the sounds of the heartbeats will get very soft and then disappear. This is your diastolic level.

Tips for Using Home Blood Pressure Monitors

During the first few weeks of using a home BP monitor, you may take your pressure several times a day. You probably will also take the pressure of other family members and friends. If your find that you get different readings each time you take your pressure, don't assume the monitor is malfunctioning. And don't think your blood pressure is necessarily gyrating out of control. Your blood pressure changes during the day, and most people's pressure will change by as much as 20 mm Hg. Here are some tips for keeping blood pressure monitoring as stress-free and accurate as possible:

♦ When you take your blood pressure at home, it will generally be lower than the readings taken in a doctor's office. The lower reading may be due to your being more relaxed. However, it can also be due to an inaccuracy in measurement or in the placement of the cuff.

♦ Don't be tempted to take your blood pressure several times within a short period. If your reading is unusual for you—either high or low—remove the cuff and relax for at least ten minutes to let the blood flow in your arm return to normal. Then take another reading.

♦ Follow your doctor's advice on how often to take your blood pressure. Once a day, at the same time every day, is often recommended. Keep a record of the day, the time the pressure is taken, and the blood pressure reading. After a few weeks, you will be able to see a pattern.

- Unless otherwise advised, take your pressure in the morning, right after you get up and use the bathroom, but before you dress and have your breakfast. You should avoid taking your pressure when eating, drinking (especially coffee, tea, cola drinks, or alcoholic drinks), exercising, sitting in a hot tub, feeling stressed, taking illegal drugs, or doing any intense or physical work.
- Use the same arm. Be sure that you put the cuff on the right way.
- Whether you use an arm cuff or wrist monitor, position your arm a little higher than waist level, at the level of your heart, with your palm up. As explained, you measure the pressure in the brachial artery, which is a blood vessel that goes from your shoulder to just below your elbow.

A lawyer friend bought his own blood pressure equipment and started taking his blood pressure at his office. He asked me to check his readings, and I found my readings to be higher than his. A physician or trained medical assistant recognizes the sounds instantly and therefore obtains a higher and more accurate reading than a novice.

On the other hand, Dr. Christopher Cottier and his associates, writing in *The Journal of the American Medical Association*, reported that for patients with labile blood pressure—those whose readings oscillated just above and just below 150/90—self-examination was very accurate.

Henry David Thoreau, the nineteenth-century essayist, suggested that each person marches to his own drummer. That may be true in some sense, but the beat of blood pressure is the same for all human beings. Listening to your own beat can improve your understanding of yourself, and help you make any needed adjustments When you take your own blood pressure you really hear and feel the sound of your own beat.

Using Blood Pressure

You now have the basic tool to evaluate how effective your drug-free efforts will be in regulating your blood pressure. It will be a continuous job to keep your blood pressure at the normal low for your age, but you can enjoy seeing your progress. In the following pages I will provide many proven tools for bringing your high blood pressure under control.

CHAPTER 4

Diastolic and Systolic Pressure —What Does Each Mean?

Watching Diastolic Pressure

When the heart is at rest, in between beats, your blood pressure falls. This is the diastolic pressure. It is represented by the number that is lower in value, written after the slash. There is a clear-cut increase in illness and death related to high diastolic pressure. Recent findings show that this also is true for high systolic pressure. The statistics that indicate these increased health risks are startling:

- If your diastolic pressure—the lowest pressure that remains within the artery when the heart is at rest—is less than 85 mm Hg and you are between ages 50 and 59, your chances of dying of a blood-pressure-related illness are 63 out of 1,000.

- If your diastolic pressure is over 104 mm Hg for the same age range, the risks of dying are greatly increased. The possibility of suffering a stroke at this age is seven times greater in people with a diastolic pressure above 104 mm Hg than in those with a diastolic pressure below 85 mm Hg.

These figures apply only to people who are not treated for hypertension or to people who are treated but whose pressure remains high. To underscore the absolute necessity for treatment, consider the following, which also refers only to people who have not received treatment.

Labile hypertensives: The term *labile* means gliding, being unsteady or easily changed. People whose diastolic blood pressure range moves from normal to high, then back to normal with readings between 80 and

100 mm Hg, have a 90 percent survival rate for the first five years after their condition is discovered.

In the past, people with labile hypertension were considered merely borderline or transient cases. Now we know that even labile hypertension poses an increased risk and frequently can lead to full-blown hypertension. In fact, even a single high pressure reading should be followed by further readings to make sure that serious disease is not developing—and if it is, to receive immediate care.

Benign hypertensives: The term *benign* in this context means the disease is mild and that the progress of the disease will probably be slow. Those people with very mild hypertension, with diastolic pressure readings greater than 89 mm Hg, have a five-year survival rate of 66 percent.

Accelerated malignant hypertensives: Malignant hypertension progresses rapidly, accompanied by severe vascular damage. Those who have this severe hypertension, with diastolic blood pressure readings above 120 mm Hg, need immediate care.

Systolic Hypertension Is Important, Too

Your blood pressure is at its greatest when the heart contracts and is pumping the blood. This is called systolic pressure. It is noted before the diastolic pressure. What role does systolic pressure play in hypertension?

The National Heart, Lung, and Blood Institute defines normal systolic pressure as a level of 150 mm Hg or lower, with a corresponding diastolic pressure of no more than 90 mm Hg. Until recently doctors assumed that systolic hypertension had little significance. Any rise in systolic pressure was simply considered a response to aging. However, now there are indications that increased systolic pressure causes harmful effects similar to those caused by diastolic hypertension.

One study found that systolic hypertension causes an increase in brain injury, heart disease, and heart failure. Medical centers are currently evaluating this finding. The central thrust of most studies is to discover whether strokes occur more often in persons with elevated systolic pressure but normal diastolic pressure than in those whose systolic pressure is not elevated. This is an important question, because an answer will tell researchers and physicians whether strokes can be prevented if people with elevated systolic pressure but normal diastolic pressure can be helped by treatment with medication.

> ### Pressure Check
>
> For the past twenty-five years, doctors have warned people about the dangers of high blood pressure. Millions of premature deaths have been averted by those who heeded these warnings. But now it seems that the message is no longer getting through: In August 1999 a national health survey showed that the incidence of high blood pressure is no longer falling at the same rate as in the past decade. Also, the incidence of stroke has started to rise. A report in the journal *Hypertension* shows that blood pressure readings in residents of affluent neighborhoods in Minnesota are 5 percent higher than they were just ten years ago.

Effect of Aging on Systolic Pressure

As you age, the systolic pressure rises, so that your pulse pressure increases; for example, a systolic pressure of 140 and a diastolic pressure of 80 equals a pulse pressure of 60—or 20 points above normal. What causes the systolic pressure to rise with age? In large part, the rise occurs because the major arteries of the body are affected by atherosclerosis, or hardening of the arteries.

Normally, each time your heart ejects its volume of blood, the major arteries of the body absorb the pressure, and the systolic pressure does not rise above 120 mm Hg. In youth, blood flows smoothly into the largest artery in the body, the aorta, which leads away from the heart. First blood flows upward from the heart toward the neck, where another artery branches off to take blood to the head and brain. Next, blood flows downward toward the rest of the body. As you age, arteries stiffen and become less elastic, so that when the heart ejects its blood volume into the artery, the artery does not expand, and the force of the ejected blood pushing against the hardened arteries increases. When this happens, systolic pressure rises beyond 120 mm Hg.

We know some factors related to hardening of the arteries, but we do not know the cause. Several medical centers have conducted studies of systolic hypertension aimed at determining whether the systolic rise in the inelastic artery is a normal response to aging, or a disease process that can and should be treated.

Older people with systolic hypertension can control their disorder with medication, but the response is slow. Diastolic hypertension responds to treatment even more slowly than does systolic hypertension. Older patients respond particularly slowly because their bodies take longer to adjust; therefore, older people should receive medication at a slower rate and over a longer period than younger people.

Anxiety and Systolic Pressure

Systolic pressure often responds to anxiety and returns to normal once the anxiety abates. I recently saw an example of this in a patient: Before her physical examination began, the patient (I'll call her Joan) had normal blood pressure of 120/80 mm Hg. But by the time the examination was completed, her blood pressure had risen to 160/80 mm Hg. Since I knew Joan, I knew she tended to be an anxious person, so I suggested she rest in the office for half an hour after her examination. When I rechecked after this short rest, Joan's pressure was back to a normal blood pressure of 120/80 mm Hg.

Diagnosing Less Common Types of Hypertension

Hypertension regardless of cause should be treated under the direction of your physician. Some of the less common causes of high blood pressure are:

Kidney disease—accounts for 5 percent

Renovascular disease (kidney or renal hypertension)—accounts for 4 percent

Narrowing of the aorta—accounts for 1 percent

The diagnosis of the type of hypertension you have cannot be done on your own. Your doctor will decide whether you have essential high blood pressure, which seems to have no apparent cause, or whether you have a specific cause for your hypertension. Your physician will probably listen carefully to what you say, since taking a medical history that is as complete as possible is an essential first step. A few simple tests may follow. In many cases a urine test will rule out the presence of kidney disease as a cause of high blood pressure. If the urine test does not indicate you have essential high blood pressure, your physician will continue looking for the source of the problem.

A small number of cases of hypertension result from endocrine disorders or from other rare conditions. All these other forms of hypertension are less common than essential hypertension, and all have the potential of cure with either medicine or surgery.

TESTS IN YOUR DOCTOR'S OFFICE

Routine tests are often part of your medical evaluation. These are some of the tests your doctor may think are suitable for you:

Urine examination, to identify inflammation of the kidneys

Blood count:

Blood urea nitrogen (BUN), to check the functioning of the kidneys

Serum electrolytes

Serum creatinine (a protein crystal), to check the functioning of the kidneys

Serum glucose (blood sugar), to check for diabetes

Serum cholesterol, triglycerides, to check for additional risk factors for atherosclerosis (thickening of the artery walls)

Renin levels in blood

Doctors may also use imaging technology—MRIs, X-rays, ultrasound scans, and so forth—to get as much information as possible for a better evaluation of your health and to address your needs.

There are also now tests to discover whether hardening of the arteries has occurred. These tests monitor wave reflections in the walls of the aorta. Wave reflections occur when the pulse waves encounter the smaller arteries that branch off the large aorta. A computer program translates the timing of the wave reflection into a number known as the augmentation index. The higher the augmentation index, the greater the stiffness of the arteries.

If you want to know more about high blood pressure, how it is measured, and the implications of the disease for your total health, you can contact the National Heart, Lung, and Blood Institute, P.O. Box 30105, Bethesda, MD 20824-0105; 301-251-1222.

CHAPTER 5

What Happens When You Learn You Have High Blood Pressure?

Just learning you have hypertension can have side effects. These side effects have absolutely nothing to do with your blood pressure. But they do have a great deal to do with you, your personality, and the way you react to unpleasant news. Learning you have hypertension can be acknowledgment of a fact, or can seem like a verdict that leaves you feeling overwhelmed. Or it can be both reactions at once, or a completely different reaction. How you deal with hypertension is as individual as the disease and your own personality.

Replace Worry and Fear with Knowledge

If you have this book, you may already know that you, or someone you care about, has high blood pressure. If you have HBP, do you feel your own self-image has been changed? Do you feel different about yourself now that you know your blood pressure is high? How vulnerable are you to the problems that are linked with hypertension? Rather than worry, let's look into the problem—not the problem of high blood pressure, but the problem of *your reaction* to high blood pressure, which may affect the progress of the disease.

"I'M SOMEONE WITH A DISEASE"

Learning that you have any disorder can trigger strong emotions. Disease is a threat to life expectancy and an uncomfortable challenge at any age. Fearful and even angry thoughts may whirl through your mind. Will your ability to work be compromised? How will other aspects of your life be affected?

Hypertension, like most other diseases, can also mean a strain on your finances. Illness is time-consuming; it requires doctor visits and, possibly, various kinds of therapy. If antihypertensive medications are called for, there is the potential of having to deal with drug-related side effects. You will be forced to review your basic life priorities and your lifestyle. People with hypertension often feel their self-esteem diminished. Clinical experience as well as many studies have shown that this kind of self-perception can inspire a variety of reactions and sometimes have serious effects. Here are some common responses:

- Some people worry more about their health than is normal or desirable. People like this see themselves in terms of their blood pressure.

- In others, finding out they are hypertensive has caused a decrease in self-esteem, well-being, and self-confidence.

- In still other people, the reaction is fatalistic. Some people see the diagnosis as a disability or a death sentence.

- Your relatives may react with fears of their own, and some people feel guilty thinking their children may inherit the tendency for hypertension.

- Some people feel increased anxiety and depression and have difficulty coping, all of which can increase the chances of serious emotional and behavioral problems.

Any of these reactions can be overwhelming. It is never easy to learn that something may be damaging your health. In working with my patients, I have always been aware of these reactions when I discuss hypertension with them. I try to be completely honest—but also to focus on how hypertension can be managed, and the many areas in which their life's pleasures are not forever denied. Good food, physical activity, independence, and a rewarding sex life are all still possible.

Many people learn they have hypertension during an examination to investigate some other complaint. Because they have had no HBP symptoms, or their symptoms seem so vague and unspecific, hearing the diagnosis comes as an unpleasant surprise. Some patients immediately ask questions; others seem to have no reaction and make no comment. I try to modify my counseling to each patient's needs and my sense of their personality, but I also know that it's best to be honest and up-front. Don't hesitate to find out as much as you can about hypertension. Ask your doctor questions if you find any information confusing.

WHAT IS YOUR REACTION?

When people learn they have hypertension they may see it as destructive to their self-image. It may conjure up memories or whispers by adults when they were a child, or of some relative with hypertension who then had a stroke and died. The net effect is instant confrontation with mortality. "How can this have happened to me?" is a typical refrain. On the other hand, many people respond to the diagnosis with optimism and a commitment to do what is necessary. These people are the ones more likely to manage the disease and live a long and healthy life.

DEFENSE MECHANISMS

Being labeled a hypertensive may inspire any one of a number of defense mechanisms. The two most common ones I've observed are:

Denial: People try to protect themselves from unpleasantness by simply refusing to acknowledge it. They wrongly feel that if they ignore the unpleasant news, the hypertension will just go away.

Displacement: Others feel that when something goes wrong, someone or something must be at fault or to blame. We should all remember that bad things do happen to good people—and blame does not lower blood pressure.

Reactions Differ

Over my decades as a physician I've met many memorable hypertension patients. Here are some stories of typical reactions to hypertension. Do any of them remind you of yourself?

Bill denies the problem: Bill was a successful author of 60 when he learned he had high blood pressure. A man who prided himself on his youthful vitality, Bill insisted that he felt fine and nothing was wrong. Bill's doctor, who tried to convince Bill of the seriousness of his condition, was ignored. Instead of following sound medical advice (and perhaps seeking false reassurance of his health), Bill started an unsupervised exercise program; six months later, he was the victim of a stroke.

Bill's is a typical case of *denial.* He felt well and refused to believe that anything could possibly be wrong. Unfortunately, many people, like Bill, reject medical findings and refuse to return to the doctor who has confronted them with the diagnosis of hypertension. Perhaps most dangerous is that denial makes people refuse any positive changes in their life.

Ann places blame: At 55, Ann developed hypertension. She had a high-pressure job and often complained about her dictatorial boss. When hypertension was diagnosed, Ann blamed her job, her boss, her phone, and even her computer. Ann's *displacement* (blaming an outside person or situation) became so intense that she had to give up her job. Later she learned that her boss would gladly have reorganized her workload and made adjustments had he known of her condition.

Ken fears history will be repeated: Ken is a physician whose father died at an early age of a massive stroke. Confronted with a diagnosis of hypertension, Ken became haunted by the fear that he would die as his father had. He felt guilty because he thought his children might be similarly afflicted. Ken became incapacitated. His reaction was extreme, but it does occur—even among physicians.

People like Bill, Ann, and Ken are intelligent and reasonable in most situations, but because HBP has so few symptoms, they choose to ignore all medical instructions. Noncompliance is another way of denying reality. I've even heard the complaint: "If the doctor hadn't told me, I'd still be okay." Saddest of all is that denial prevents people from making the basic changes that can actually increase their vitality, feeling of well-being—and even their looks. I wish I could convince these patients they can do something!

Here are the stories of two other patients, Irene and George. Both eventually would manage their HBP and enjoy life, although one did so only reluctantly.

Irene worries about everything: When Irene had the flu, she coughed and sneezed so often she had a nosebleed. After several tests, her physician told Irene that her blood pressure was elevated. Irene insisted that she felt fine and was not disturbed by the diagnosis. But Irene soon became worried about her general health and sought constant *reassurance,* which made her feel better and allowed her to embark on a successful treatment regimen. Medical reassurance is often essential to the emotional stability of the hypertension patient.

George makes changes: When the diagnosis of essential hypertension was confirmed, George immediately embarked on a self-help program. He joined a health club, and with the help of a qualified health care profes-sional exercised daily and swam three times a week. The changes in George's dietary habits were also striking: He had enjoyed cholesterol-laden, heavily salted foods such as bacon. But after the diagnosis, George ate a healthful, nutritionally rich, balanced diet. When we had dinner, George ordered broiled fish and even suggested we divide the serving be-tween us. George lost excess weight and kept an ideal weight.

George decided to take control of his life and deal with high blood pres-sure by making changes in his lifestyle. What he did for himself was a form of *compensation,* and it was remarkable. The reward: George's blood pres-sure came down, and he felt great. He told me, "I feel better since I learned I was sick; I guess it's because I'm doing something about it."

Sir William Osler, the famed physician and former head of the Johns Hopkins Medical School, said, "Someone with a chronic illness who is forced to take good care of himself will outlive the healthy person who does not." This concept is especially true for hypertensive patients who respond to their diagnosis by showing self-control and making changes in the way they live.

THE EFFECTS OF SELF-IMAGE ON HEALTH

My observations are similar to those of physicians throughout the world. Finding out that you have a serious disease is always traumatic, and some patients see themselves in terms of that disease, even without any symp-toms.

The possible dangers of being labeled hypertensive were explored in the British medical journal *The Lancet* several years ago. In a study, seventy-one people were told they had hypertension when in fact they did not. These volunteers responded to this news by becoming depressed, hostile, and feeling ill. At the same time, members of a control group who did not have hypertension were told their blood pressure was normal. They re-sponded by feeling good, more physically fit, and happier.

In another study to determine the effects of labeling, four groups were examined:

1. People who were labeled hypertensive and were hypertensive.

2. Hypertensives who did not know they had HBP, and who later discov-ered their condition.

3. People who were labeled hypertensive but actually were not.

4. People who knew they did not have hypertension.

The people in groups 1 and 3 suffered greater psychological distress than those in groups 2 and 4. Conclusion: Learning you have hypertension may cause strong emotional reactions, even emotional problems.

Hypertension on the Job

People with HBP are everywhere; they are a large segment of the workforce. Although the practice of treating people at their workplace is not new, unfortunately it is still not widely accepted. Obviously, people treated at work are less likely to be absent than those who must seek treatment elsewhere.

If you are an employer, you should recognize there are some practical reasons for helping hypertensive employees. Since many hypertensive employees are among the most productive people, it is just good sense and good business to keep such employees feeling their best. When a worker has a problem, he or she should be examined on the spot, and unless the problem is serious, the worker should stay on the job.

CORPORATE/CAREER SIDE EFFECTS

Many people are worried about the career impact of letting an employer know that they have high blood pressure. Employees are also worried about their health care coverage, and how high blood pressure will affect their premiums. But it is more important to attend to your health. If you are hypertensive, find out what resources are available at your workplace or nearby, and make use of them—even if it means just checking your blood pressure. And if you work for yourself, as so many people do, treat yourself as a valued employee.

"I'M SICK BECAUSE I THINK I'M SICK"

Absenteeism from work is higher among people aware they have hypertension than among those unaware of their condition. Labeling and the absenteeism linked to it can be present even in someone not taking medication. Absenteeism from work cannot automatically be attributed to side effects of medication; it sometimes may be an emotional result of labeling.

Knowledge and understanding in care and treatment can often prevent or reverse this increased absenteeism. For example, a patient called my office early one morning complaining of a headache; he thought it best to skip work. I was familiar with his hypertension and advised him to "take two aspirin and go to work." Giving him that advice would have been fraught with danger if I had not been familiar with his medical status. (Headaches sometimes are the forerunner of a stroke, in which case telling him to go to work would have been very bad advice.) Just to be on the safe side, I asked him to stop at my office when he left work that evening. When the patient arrived, a check of his blood pressure indicated it was within the safe limits. My worried patient said his headache disappeared soon after taking the aspirin. Medical reassurance can often overcome or reduce the fears of hypertensives.

The Type A Personality as a Factor in High Blood Pressure

As you can see, your personality is a key factor in how you react to HBP. You've probably noticed that some people—so-called type A personalities—seem more fast-moving and aggressive than others. Are you one of those people? Here are a few questions that will help you recognize if you are:

- Do you become frustrated and angry when you have to wait for stoplights, elevators, or slow transactions?
- Do you set tough goals for yourself at home, in sports, at recreation, as well as at work?
- Do you become impatient and finish other people's sentences? Do you tend to leap to conclusions before you hear the details?
- Do you always want to do more, achieve more, have more—in less time?

If you answered yes to any of these questions, your personality may be a factor in your hypertension. While our society may reward this behavior, our bodies, which were developed eons before airplanes, phones, and six-lane highways, do not respond with rewards. There is little hard evidence to link type A personalities with hypertension and studies are inconclusive, but anecdotal evidence makes me feel the personality factor cannot be ignored.

What happens when high-pressure people (type A personalities) are labeled hypertensive? I've seen some type A people make a complete reversal of behavior patterns; they stop pressuring themselves and sometimes they even cut back on work and social engagements and become more relaxed. Others become even more driven, impatient, and anxious because they feel their time is running out and they will be unable to achieve their goals.

The Renin Reaction

When treatment doesn't seem to control hypertension, some patients may have more intense emotions than do most people. Reactive high blood pressure occurs when the body reacts to stressful or threatening situations by releasing a kidney protein/enzyme called renin. Renin works in part by stimulating a portion of the nervous system by raising the blood pressure, and a feeling of tension may result from this stimulation. A substantial group of hypertensives have high renin levels. It is possible that those with high renin levels are more difficult to treat. Our knowledge of the exact role of renin in the cause and prolongation of hypertension is still limited, but a group of drugs called renin inhibitors is now available. For more about emotional triggers to HBP, see Chapter 25, "Stress and Hypertension."

Labels and Treatment

Determining the effect of labeling on hypertensive persons is important because hypertension can get worse just because you know you have it. It is particularly tricky in those whose hypertension is so near normal levels that medication is not needed or even may be harmful. The doctor's dilemma at this stage is to decide whether it is better not to tell such persons that they have hypertension, or to tell them because they should be under medical care. Obviously, people with more severe hypertension *must* know about their condition as a first step in treatment.

Whether you have hypertension or simply want to try to avoid the disorder, a good start is to learn all you can about high blood pressure. It is also wise to understand the forms of treatment available and the changes in your lifestyle that will help you manage the disease. If you have even mild hypertension, you should become a partner with your physician to aid in its therapy. Knowledge is power.

Today, because health fairs and blood pressure machines are often locally available, more people are having their blood pressure tested and take active measures in its control. But many others either never bother to check their blood pressure or don't follow their doctor's orders. Follow-through includes making lifestyle changes and having your progress checked, since your treatment needs probably will change over time. Only by taking charge of your health will you get the most from your treatment. So start now to lower your high blood pressure, and treat your blood pressure as if your life depended on that treatment. It may.

CHAPTER 6

Do It for Yourself

Now you know how to check your own blood pressure, and you understand the dangers of high blood pressure. What more can you do to improve your health and enjoy your life? You must be your own first line of defense against hypertension. Use this book as a tool to help you plan your campaign to lower your blood pressure and to win the battle against this potentially harmful disease.

In 1984, the *New York Times* carried a front-page story about new federal government guidelines for the treatment of high blood pressure. Prepared by the National Heart, Lung, and Blood Institute, the recommendations emphasized nondrug treatments, such as diet, exercise, and behavior modifications. Now, nearly two decades later, despite amazing medical advances, those recommendations are just as valid. In fact, more and more people are taking control of their own health by learning how they can change some small aspect of their life to improve their total well-being. We are also becoming more interested in the medical treatments used in ancient history and those of various other cultures. If they've worked for others, why not see if they are valid for us?

"We are responding to a lot of underlying concern about the toxicity of antihypertensive drugs and their side effects," said Dr. Harriet P. Dustan, director of cardiovascular research at the University of Alabama. She added: "For instance, there is growing appreciation of the fact that obesity and hypertension are closely related. You may be able to control mild hypertension with weight reduction."

Doctors now focus on prevention, recommending ways to eliminate or change risk factors that you can control, as well as treating serious medical events. Noninvasive lifestyle therapies are to be "pursued aggressively" in treating the mildest cases of hypertension. For more severe cases, the medical experts suggest that nondrug therapies be used as an adjunct in treatment to reduce the quantity of medicines needed.

The Advantages of Nondrug Therapy

Antihypertensive drugs all have side effects, some of which are minor and hardly noticeable, while others can compound existing health problems. *Note: You should never stop taking blood pressure medications or change your therapy program without consulting your doctor.*

Here's an all-too-typical tale of the relationship between lifestyle and high blood pressure. Forty-five-year-old John, recently divorced and worried about money, is told by his doctor that he has early hypertension. John is unperturbed, even though his parents suffered from hypertension. After work, he usually drives his 200-pound body through heavy rush-hour traffic. During the difficult drive home John dwells on the frustrations of his job. He feels his boss pressures him to work harder and harder, without either appreciation or compensation. John often thinks his job is killing him.

A two-pack-a-day chain-smoker, John often eats at a local fast food restaurant. His favorite meal consists of French fries, a bacon cheeseburger, and two large Cokes. At home, John relaxes in an easy chair; after a few beers, he falls asleep. Sometimes he is so tired he avoids meeting friends or even going to a movie.

After a time, John develops headaches, which he passes off as just part of daily living. Eventually, severe nosebleeds send him to a doctor. His blood pressure is quite high. John is put on medication to control his hypertension, but he soon has trouble functioning sexually, so he stops taking his medication. John has his first stroke at age 46.

If you see yourself in John's story, or if you answer yes to any of the following questions, it is time—perhaps past time—for you to make some changes in your lifestyle. You'll be exchanging some counterproductive habits for some health-building ones.

- ◆ Do you tend to ignore warnings? Do you listen to what your doctor tells you and then promptly forget his or her suggestions once you leave the office?

- Do you drive yourself to excel, to do a better job faster than anyone else? Do you worry that others may be gaining on you at work?

- Do you go over and over annoying things until you are in a rage? Do you become furious if you are stuck in traffic, or are forced to wait in a slow-moving line?

- Do you salt your food before you even taste it? Do you crave salty foods?

- Do you enjoy eating and drinking too much to worry that your weight is slowly mounting?

- Do you think that exercise is for jocks and that you get enough for the average person? When you do exert yourself, do you find that you are immediately exhausted?

If you answered yes to many or most of these questions, you may find that you are headed on a dangerous course.

High Blood Pressure and Lifestyle

John's case history is exaggerated—but only slightly. I've invented it to demonstrate that you are not only what you eat but also what you think and what you do. There are a number of things you should do to minimize the chances of getting high blood pressure or to reduce the risks if you already have hypertension.

Control your HBP by eating a nutritious diet, counting your calories, and keeping a healthy weight. A healthy diet is low in salt intake and high in minerals and other nutrients. Stress and anxiety can do irreparable harm to your body and also tend to increase consumption of tobacco and alcohol. Exercise can dissipate stress; being active every day is important. Most of all, if you have high blood pressure, you must obtain medical care and follow treatment.

The remaining units of this book consist of information about HBP and programs for you to consider and follow. They are based on therapies I've developed over several decades of working with patients, and they are also recommended by the medical experts who have studied hypertension. Weight control, salt reduction, alcohol and tobacco restriction, relaxation techniques, exercise, and many other strategies are explored. But before you begin, I urge you first to talk to your own doctor. *Don't embark on self-medication.* You must involve yourself in your own health care, but involvement and participation does not exclude the professionals.

Working with Your Health Team

Once your learn that you have HBP, you'll probably start a program to manage your blood pressure and to reduce it. Your doctor and you will be partners in that program, and together you can accomplish much more than you can alone.

After you and your doctor have begun therapy and have scheduled regular office visits, some problems with keeping on your therapy program may arise. Here are some tips for working with your doctor to keep your blood pressure in the normal range.

1. Keep your appointments with your doctor and other health care professionals. This will help your team keep records of your progress, and to monitor the effectiveness of any drugs that are prescribed. Your doctor will probably take your blood pressure in the office and discuss your pressure numbers with you. Make sure you understand the meaning of the numbers.

2. Talk about your goal for lowering your pressure. (Doctors like to see patients improve.) If you have any questions about your doctor's instructions, this is the time to ask. Don't hesitate, no matter how small or seemingly insignificant they may seem; your concerns and questions can be important.

3. If your doctor has any handouts, ask for them. And if you have questions about any written material—including this book—ask for clarification. Remember, your physician knows you better than any book! When your doctor gives you directions, repeat them back in your own words, so your physician can be sure you understand them.

4. Your doctor expects you to adhere to your program and to work toward lowering your pressure and improving health. Expect to slip from time to time—but keep moving toward your goal. Keep following medical advice about diet and exercise. Work to avoid or deal with stress. Make the necessary changes in your life habits.

5. If you do take HBP medications, take them as directed. Tell your doctor if you feel any side effects, no matter how trivial they may seem to you. How a medication makes you feel affects how you adhere to the medication program.

6. If your program works and you see a downward trend in your blood pressure, enjoy your progress. Both you and your physician can feel proud. Seek reinforcement and support for the program you and your

doctor decide on from friends and family, as well as from other health care providers.

Monitoring your blood pressure is a way to head off the problems of hypertension. Of all the ailments you might have, hypertension is the one most affected by your lifestyle, so monitoring your lifestyle is essential. Let's get started!

PART II

Your Diet

or Your Life

What should you eat to get healthy and stay healthy? Food, like medicine, contributes to our health. Sometimes advice is confusing. But a little knowledge can help you select foods that will reduce or even eliminate reliance on traditional drug therapies—and let you enjoy every meal and snack.

CHAPTER 7

The Truth About Salt

Salt has an exciting past. Once salt was scarce and almost as precious as gold. The word *salary* comes from *salt,* since many of the thousands of Roman soldiers were paid in a measure of salt. Modern technology, however, has made salt readily available and affordable.

Salt, or sodium chloride, is essential for maintaining the body's blood volume and controlling the movement of fluids in and out of the cells. Sodium is the main component of the body's extracellular fluids and it helps carry nutrients to the cells. Sodium helps to regulate other body functions, such as blood pressure and fluid volume. It also works on the lining of blood vessels to keep the pressure balance normal. Sodium is vital for transmitting nerve impulses and in metabolizing proteins and carbohydrates to produce energy. The chloride part of the salt molecule helps in maintaining the body's normal acid balance and is necessary for some enzymes to do their work. Here are examples of sodium at work:

- Blood: Sodium helps to maintain the blood's pH (acid/alkaline) balance.
- Digestive system: Too much salt causes the stomach to make too much hydrochloric acid.
- Nerves: The transmission of nerve impulses depends partly on sodium.
- Metabolism: Sodium assists the cells in your intestines in absorbing food.
- Muscles: Without sodium, your muscles could not contract.

Salt Makes It Happen

Food anthropologists think our enjoyment of salty food dates back about eight thousand years to when human beings went from gathering food and hunting to cultivating crops and domesticating animals. To survive, ancient people needed to preserve food for the winter. One available way was to salt it; salt cuts down on bacterial growth. Salt has other enticements: It reduces the boiling point of water, helps heat penetrate cooking foods, and conditions dough in baked products. Salt adds flavor, and some foods, like cheese, require salt for their formation. The real advantage may be that it enhances all the other flavors—even sweetness.

Salt is one of the four taste categories—salty, sweet, sour, and bitter. We start our taste for a high salt level as babies. Mother tastes the food and judges it according to *her* taste level, which then becomes the infant's starting taste level. (Note: Many baby foods now advertise that they are low-salt because people are becoming more aware of the power of salt.) Salt has a certain addictive quality. As you increase your salt intake, your taste buds become accustomed to new levels of salt concentration; to taste of salt again, you must constantly increase the amount you use.

If It Tastes So Good, How Can It Be Bad?

Doctors have been suspicious of the effects of too much salt for a long time: Physicians in China in 2500 B.C. warned their patients that using too much salt would cause the pulse to "harden." Dr. Jeffrey Cutler, director of the Clinical Applications and Prevention Program of the National Heart, Lung, and Blood Institute, points out, "The conclusion is still there: The higher the salt intake the higher the prevalence of hypertension." If you still have any doubts, a study in 1995, with results published in the professional journal *Nature Medicine,* shows that chimpanzees, the species closest to humans, will develop high blood pressure when their diet is too high in salt. And in a 1993 study, baby rats were fed diets naturally high in salt. The rats were examined in two studies: Within two weeks of starting the high-salt diet, they had elevated blood pressure.

Healthy kidney function can rid the body of excess salt, but that happens at the expense of losing calcium. For women, and even older men, some studies suggest that this depletion of calcium may eventually be linked to the bone disease osteoporosis, in which long-term calcium loss causes bones to weaken and break easily. Salt also creates excess strain on the heart, and heart failure can be triggered or aggravated by a diet high in salt.

For many years, it was generally thought that people could salt to suit their taste without adverse effects; the body would simply pass the excess salt out of its system. We now know that this is incorrect. Some people respond to excess salt by developing hypertension.

But doesn't everyone need some salt? Yes, but no one needs salt beyond the very basic daily requirement. Almost everyone should cut down on salt intake. For people with any degree of hypertension—be it mild or severe— salt intake must be reduced.

To Salt . . . or Not to Salt

Cutting back on salt will not cure high blood pressure or even be an adequate total treatment. But for most people with mild hypertension, or those who simply want to avoid any blood pressure problems, a reduction in their salt intake will result in lower blood pressure readings. Even those who need medication to treat their high blood pressure will respond better to drugs when they follow a low-salt diet.

Laura's Story

Although Laura was a professional dietitian, she paid no attention to her own diet. She often ate fast food and other "convenience" foods. When Laura became troubled by persistent nosebleeds, she tried to ignore the problem, but the bleeding became intense, forcing her to consult a physician. The nosebleeds were caused by high blood pressure. After examining Laura's diet, her physician recommended a drastic cut in her salt intake.

Shaken by the severity of her symptoms and by the diagnosis, Laura decided to practice what she preached as a dietitian. She placed herself on a 1 gram (1,000 milligrams, or ½ teaspoon) sodium diet. She banished salt from the dining table, used no salt in cooking, and avoided any foods that had a high sodium content. For a while, nothing tasted right, but the adjustment to the loss of salt became easier when she noted that her blood pressure was going down. At her last checkup, Laura's blood pressure was normal.

The body can lose sodium by a number of routes other than in the urine. Sweating, vomiting, and diarrhea can also produce dramatic sodium loss. For people who lose too much potassium from taking diuretics, reducing salt intake will help to retain this vital mineral. Reducing salt intake is important for many people. The body has a wonderful system to regulate body sodium. The goal of a low-sodium diet is to push this regulation system toward one end of its range, without pushing it too far. A low-sodium diet can be overdone, however. The level of sodium intake should be decided in consultation with your physician or nutritionist.

HOW MUCH IS ENOUGH, BUT NOT TOO MUCH?

Americans consume too much salt. One teaspoon has 2 grams (2,000 milligrams) of sodium. Americans now consume between 2.3 and 6.9 grams daily, or about 3 teaspoons of salt. This is three times more than we actually need. The National Research Council maintains that a safe and adequate daily sodium intake is about 1,100 to 3,300 milligrams (mg) for adults.

High-salt diet: 4,000–6,000 mg/day (2 to 3 teaspoons)

Normal salt diet: 1,500–3,000 mg/day (¾ to 1½ teaspoons)

Low-salt diet: 500–1,000 mg/day (¼ to ½ teaspoon)

Extremely low-salt diet: 200–500 mg/day (just a pinch)

How much is really enough? It is difficult to determine the exact minimal amount of sodium your body needs daily to function. After reading and studying many reports, I believe the best estimate is somewhere below 500 milligrams of sodium a day—that is, about one-quarter teaspoon. Once I became aware of the small amount the body really needs each day, the amount of salt many people actually consume seems even higher.

The salt content of many common foods is astonishingly high. The list on pages 314–15 provides an overview of the quantity of salt in the food and drink most of us consume. You will find some surprises. For example, a 6-ounce glass of tomato juice has 659 milligrams of sodium, about the minimum recommended daily amount.

Sodium Where You Least Suspect

Sodium chloride isn't the only form of sodium that may affect your blood pressure. Many people with high blood pressure are sensitive to other

Salt in a Teaspoon		
⅛ teaspoon of salt	=	250 milligrams of sodium
¼ teaspoon of salt	=	500 milligrams of sodium
½ teaspoon of salt	=	1,000 milligrams of sodium
¾ teaspoon of salt	=	1,500 milligrams of sodium
1 teaspoon of salt	=	2,000 milligrams of sodium

sodium compounds. These people are what is known as sodium-sensitive and apparently have a genetic predisposition to high blood pressure. They need to be aware of all sodium compounds that may be used to process foods:

- Baking soda (sodium bicarbonate) is used to leaven breads and cakes; it is sometimes taken for indigestion.

- Baking powder is a mixture of baking soda, starch, and an acid, used in quick breads and cake.

- Monosodium glutamate (MSG) is used to enhance flavor in restaurant cooking and in many packaged, canned, and frozen foods.

- Sodium alginate is used in making chocolate milk and ice cream into smoothie mixtures.

- Sodium benzoate is used to preserve many condiments, such as relishes and sauces.

- Sodium hydroxide is used to soften and loosen skins of some canned or frozen fruits and vegetables.

- Sodium nitrate is used to cure meats and sausages.

- Sodium sulfite is used to preserve dried fruits.

SALT BY ANY OTHER NAME IS SODIUM

What is the difference between salt and sodium? Salt is a form of sodium. Should you look for salt or sodium on the nutrition label? Look for sodium. It is the chemical. Salt is the name of the product that is 40 percent sodium and 60 percent chloride. To find out how much salt is in your food, turn to the chart "Sodium in Foods," on pages 314–15. This chart has been produced by a team of nutritionists and dietitians to guide people with

---

Did You Know?

One tablespoon of chili sauce on your hamburger adds 227 mg of sodium.

Drench sushi in soy sauce and you'll take in 1,029 mg of sodium.

Eat a frankfurter (639 mg) on a bun (202 mg) with sauerkraut (one-eighth cup, for 179 mg) and you'll consume 1,020 mg of sodium. Add a dill pickle slice for another 232 mg to bring the total to 1,252 milligrams.

HBP; it was developed in 1993. A new chart is developed every ten years, or when food tastes and markets change.

Salt quickly adds up. But there is good news: Fresh meat, poultry, fruits, and vegetables are low in sodium. Many people think that pork should not appear on a low-salt diet. But fresh pork usually has no more sodium than do beef or poultry. Here are a few guidelines to help you keep dishes low in sodium.

LOW-SODIUM FOOD CHOICES

If you consume more sodium than you want to, consider choosing these lower sodium alternative foods. For labeled items, check the percentage of a normal daily sodium requirement of about 2,000–2,500 milligrams. Try to select foods that provide 5 percent or less of the daily requirement. Here are some suggestions:

◆ Instead of smoked, cured, and canned meat, fish, and poultry, choose unsalted fresh or frozen beef, lamb, pork, fish, and poultry. Bacon, sausage, and some barbecues are high in salt.

◆ Instead of cheese and regular peanut butter, choose low-sodium cheese and unsalted peanut butter.

◆ Instead of salted soda crackers, choose unsalted tortillas.

◆ Instead of canned and dehydrated soups, broths, and bouillon, choose low-sodium varieties.

◆ Instead of canned vegetables, choose fresh or frozen vegetables.

◆ Instead of salted snacks, choose unsalted tortilla chips, pretzels, potato chips, popcorn, and rice cakes.

The 9 Highest and the 9 Lowest Sodium Foods

Note: All values are in milligrams of sodium for a 3.5-ounce food portion.

EAT IT UP:

Apple, 1	Asparagus, 1	Banana, 1
Corn grits, 1	Cranberry juice, 1	Honey, 5
Nuts (in shells), 1	Noodles, dry, 5	Potatoes, baked or boiled, 2–6

PASS IT BY:

Bacon, 2,000	Bouillon cubes, 24,000	Cereals, commercial, 700–1,000
Cheese, processed, 1,190	Olives, green, 2,400	Rye wafers, 885
Pizza, cheese, 750	Salad dressing, 700–1,300	Tomato ketchup, 1,042

Here's a flavorful tip one of my patients shared with me: If food tastes bland, try chewing it more thoroughly. Chewing breaks down food, allowing more molecules to interact with the taste receptors in the mouth. It may also help to alternate one food with a bite of another food. The flavor is stronger in the first bite than the following ones.

More Salt-saving Strategies

The first step in reducing salt in your diet is to remove the salt shaker from the table and to keep it off. This is not easy, but it is essential. The next step is to estimate how much salt you now consume each day. Start a daily salt evaluation using Appendix 1, Sodium in Foods. List all the foods you've eaten, the approximate size of each portion, and the amount of salt used with every dish. List everything you ate for every meal: breakfast, lunch, dinner, and snacks, as well as every beverage you drank. Once you have listed your sodium/salt intake for a few days, you have an idea of where you should start cutting, and how much salt must be cut from your diet.

READING LABELS

The National Labeling and Education Act of 1990 and regulations from the Food and Drug Administration of the U.S. Department of Agriculture have made life easier for food buyers and dieters. Under these regulations consumers can see:

Nutrition information appears in the table headed "Nutrition Facts," which is usually on the side or back of the package. Nutrition information will also be available in stores near displays of fresh food, fruits, and vegetables.

The Percentage (%) Daily Values tells consumers at a glance the levels of important nutrients in food and how those amounts fit into a daily diet.

Serving sizes closely reflect the amount people might actually eat (who can eat one teaspoon of ice cream or 3 potato chips?).

Strictly defined nutrient content claims like "low-sodium" or "salt-free." This means when you see such a claim, you can believe it.

WHAT DO THOSE LABEL WORDS MEAN?

Food products should be labeled in a way that will help us control our salt and sodium intake. Most people prefer the information by serving than by weight, especially in grams. The guidelines for this labeling are set by the government, but the *Federal Register* has already suggested the following labels for sodium and salt:

Sodium:

Sodium-free: less than 5 mg of sodium per serving.

Very low sodium: 35 mg or less per serving of about 2 tablespoons or less.

Light sodium: at least 50 percent less than in the average similar food product.

Reduced sodium: at least 25 percent less per serving than in the average similar food product.

Salt (sodium chloride):

Salt-free: no sodium or salt.

Lightly salted: at least 50 percent less salt than in the average similar food product.

Unsalted: no salt added during processing.

Here is a sample label. Notice the amount of sodium listed. It says that a serving of spaghetti sauce provides about 10 percent of your daily allowance. If you know that, you can make adjustments in the other foods you eat during the day. Knowledge is power—especially when you cut down on your salt intake.

Nutrition Facts

Serving Size: ½ cup (125 g)
Servings Per Container about 3½

Amount Per Serving

Calories 50	Calories from Fat 10

	% Daily Value*
Total Fat 1g	2%
Saturated Fat 0g	0%
Cholesterol 0mg	0%
Sodium 250mg	10%
Potassium 530mg	15%
Total Carbohydrate 9g	3%
Dietary Fiber 1g	4%
Sugars 7g	
Protein 2g	

Vitamin A 10%	•	Vitamin C 25%
Calcium 2%	•	Iron 10%

* Percent Daily Values are based on a 2,000 calorie diet. Your daily values may be higher or lower depending on your calorie needs:

	Calories:	2,000	2,500
Total Fat	Less than	65g	80g
Sat Fat	Less than	20g	25g
Cholesterol	Less than	300mg	300mg
Sodium	Less than	2,400mg	2,400mg
Potassium		3,500mg	3,500mg
Total Carbohydrate		300g	375g
Dietary Fiber		25g	30g

What Is Safe?

Those who make unusual demands on their body's salt supply (because of very hot weather or profuse sweating) should be especially aware of the minimal body need for salt. For example, you can safely reduce sodium intake to 1,100 to 3,500 mg a day. Although this is considered a safe level, it is still quite a bit more salt than is actually good for most of us. It is believed that excess salt is usually passed out of the body, and that people who are salt-sensitive develop high blood pressure. If you exercise, you need to replace the salt lost in sweat. The total amount of needed salt is very small, and the kidneys correct the loss with ease.

People who exercise when the temperature is high, or athletes who are very active and sweat a great deal, may also have to watch their salt intake closely because salt is lost in their sweat. However, people who take salt tablets to make up this difference may develop a form of heat exhaustion from an overdose of salt. Too much salt in your bloodstream can lead to the formulation of blood clots, which can cause serious complications. An overdose of salt can be dangerous, and in some cases it can be fatal. During hot weather, or during times of stress—when you perspire a great

---

Herbal Zest

Basil	Marjoram	Sage
Bay leaf	Mint	Savory
Chives	Oregano	Tarragon
Fennel	Rosemary	Thyme
Allspice	Ginger	Paprika
Cinnamon	Mace	Pepper (black, red)
Cloves	Mustard	Curry
Nutmeg	Saffron	Turmeric
Almond	Orange	Strawberry
Lemon	Peppermint	Raspberry
Maple	Rum	Vanilla
Anise	Dill	Sesame
Caraway	Poppy seed	Cocoa
Fresh horseradish	Onion	Leeks
Orange peel	Green pepper	Lemon juice
Parsley		

deal—you may want to monitor your salt intake and your blood pressure closely.

The degree of salt restriction can vary with the level of high blood pressure, the health of your heart, and the state of your kidneys. Consult your doctor before you undertake a severely reduced salt diet.

Spicing Your Life

If you think that a low-salt diet must be a bland diet, think again. There is more taste per teaspoon in spices than most of us are aware of. I recommend you go to your food store and select a small sample of some herbs. Smell the bottles or cans, and you'll be able to tell if you enjoy the aromas; be guided by your nose. (The smell of herbs is often thought to be part of their flavor.) "Herbal Zest" gives a list of the most popular spices; below is a guide to how most people use them.

SOME SALT-FREE FLAVOR COMBINATIONS

To reduce salt in your diet, try these combinations of flavors and spices:

Chicken: cranberry sauce, ginger (fresh or canned), onion, paprika, parsley, sage, tarragon, thyme, tomato

Turkey: cranberries, rosemary

Fish: basil, bay leaf, dill, garlic powder, green pepper, lemon juice, mushrooms, onion, paprika, rosemary, savory, tomato

Beef: basil, bay leaf, dry mustard, garlic powder, green pepper, marjoram, onion, oregano, pepper, sage, thyme, tomato, vinegar

Lamb: cinnamon, curry, dill, garlic (fresh or powder), mint, mint jelly, pineapple rings, rosemary, thyme

Pork: apples, applesauce, caraway, garlic, onion, sage

Eggs: curry, dill, dry mustard, green pepper, fruit jelly, mushrooms, oregano, paprika, parsley, tomato

Veal: bay leaf, currant jelly, curry, garlic, ginger, mace, marjoram, mushrooms, oregano, paprika, spiced apricots or peaches

Asparagus: basil, caraway, lemon juice, thyme

Beans (green or wax): basil, dill, lemon juice, nutmeg, onion, oregano, rosemary, savory, sesame seeds (toasted), turmeric, unsalted toasted almonds

Broccoli: basil, lemon juice, oregano, tarragon, dill, paprika, parsley

Corn: chives, green pepper, tomato

Peas: chives, green pepper, mint, mushrooms, onion

Potatoes: chives, green pepper, mace, onion, paprika, parsley, rosemary

Squash (summer): basil, onion, oregano, pepper

Squash (winter): brown sugar, cinnamon, ginger, mace

Sweet potatoes: apples, cinnamon, nutmeg, orange juice, sugar (brown or white)

Tomatoes: basil, onion, oregano, sugar, vinegar

WHAT IS "NO-SALT SALT"?

Almost every supermarket carries products touted as "no-salt seasoners." They promise saltlike flavor without the sodium chloride content. The label usually says the product contains potassium chloride, potassium bar-

---

Hot 'n' Spicy Seasoning

¼ cup paprika

2 tablespoons oregano

2 teaspoons chili powder

1 teaspoon ground black pepper

½ teaspoon ground red pepper

½ teaspoon dry mustard

Mix all of the above in a bowl and store in an airtight container. This seasoning can be used on meat, poultry, or fish. Sprinkle on the food and cook as usual. It can also be used to make croutons and flavored bread crumbs, or it can be sprinkled over unsalted crackers for a snack. A small amount of Hot 'n' Spicy mixed with white vinegar and a very small quantity of olive oil, shaken in a small bottle, can be used as a salad dressing.

Another no-salt seasoning mix is given in the recipe section, on page 284. It's convenient to have both recipes mixed and available.

biturates, and other items. They make their sodium-free claim because they contain less than 10 milligrams of sodium per 100 grams of the food. But these products are not always a solution to your flavor problem: Potassium is similar in many ways to sodium. While potassium can taste similar to sodium chloride, it has been known to create problems for people with kidney disease, as well as life-threatening heart rhythm disturbances. If you have any serious health problems, salt substitutes with potassium should not be used without your doctor's approval.

If you'd like to create your own no-salt seasoning, here is a good starting recipe. Try making a small amount; taste it and use it in several of your favorite dishes. If you do not like the flavor, adjust the recipe to your own liking.

Salty Water

Studies have shown that municipal water supplies can contain from 5 to more than 1,000 milligrams of sodium for every liter of water. (A liter is a little more than a quart.) The 1,000 milligrams is more than the suggested daily sodium intake. It's about the same amount of salt as in a dill pickle. The water from private wells can be just as salt-laden. In some parts of the country, wells also contain about 1,000 milligrams of sodium per liter.

Although most water systems are much lower in salt, daily use of such water for cooking and drinking can result in your getting more sodium than you want. If you are serious about cutting your sodium intake, investigate the many water filters available on the market. Some can be part of an under-the-sink filtration system that also rids your water of other contaminants.

BEWARE WATER SOFTENERS

Many water softeners replace unwanted hard water chemicals with sodium. Drink a glass of water that has been through your water softener, and then drink an untreated glass of water. You may be able to taste the salt in the softened water.

Check the Labels of Over-the-Counter Medications

List the medications you are taking; some may be very high in salt. For example, laxatives, cough medications, antibiotics, alkalizers, painkillers, antacids, and sedatives all contain a great deal of sodium. Here is a sample of sodium-rich over-the-counter medications.

Rolaids (1 tablet): 53 milligrams

Alka-Seltzer (2 tablets): 521 milligrams

Bromo-Seltzer: 717 milligrams

Here is a list of commonly used over-the-counter medications that are sodium-free. But check all labels just to be sure.

Aspirin (read label*)	Sudafed
Comtrex	Ecotrin
Milk of Magnesia	Sine-Off
Vanquish	CoTylenol
Sine-Aid	Pepto-Bismol
Nytol	Triaminic products
Excedrin	Tylenol
Bufferin	Contac
Coricidin	Sominex
Robitussin-DM	

*Note: According to the Joint National Committee on High Blood Pressure, nonsteroid anti-inflammatory agents, such as aspirin, can keep diuretics, which reduce the volume of fluid in the blood, from doing their job. If you take a medication to lower your blood pressure, check with your

---

The Salt Institute Doesn't Agree

In September of 1996 the Salt Institute filed a Citizen's Petition asking the U.S. Food and Drug Administration (FDA) to rescind its permission for food manufacturers to make health claims in nutrition labels on products about the relationship between sodium and hypertension (high blood pressure). But in December of 1996 the Salt Institute withdrew its petition. Experts don't always agree: Some experts believe obesity may be the culprit behind high blood pressure, others point to salt. It is generally agreed that reducing weight as well as reducing salt intake makes good sense.

physician before you take any other medication, including any over-the-counter drug.

Sources of Information About a Salt-Free Diet

Bookstores and libraries have many books about cooking with less salt. Newspapers and magazines often offer low-salt recipes. When eating out, choose items that are less likely to have large amounts of salt added. Some restaurants will prepare low-sodium meals if asked. For more information about salt in your diet, contact Department of Health and Human Services, Food and Drug Administration, HFI-40, Rockville, MD 20857; http://www.fda.gov.

The Consumer Information Center has free copies of *Sodium: Think About It* and *A Word About Low Sodium Diets*. Write to the CIC at P.O. Box 100, Pueblo, CO 81009; http://www.pueblo.gsa.gov.

For many people, following a salt-restricted diet need not be difficult. You may find that reaching for fresh fruit rather than a salty snack will become automatic in a few weeks.

CHAPTER 8

Obesity Is a Hypertension Issue

Have you noticed how big we're getting? And, I don't mean in height! Does weight affect hypertension? It certainly does.

Everyone needs a certain amount of body fat for stored energy, heat insulation, shock absorption, and even for cosmetic reasons. But many Americans are at risk for a wide range of health problems because they are obese. As a rule, women have more body fat than men, so doctors generally agree that men with more than 25 percent body fat and women with more than 30 percent body fat are obese. The difference between being plump, overweight, and obese is a matter of degree.

What Is Obesity?

Overweight refers to an excess amount of body weight that includes all tissues—muscle, bone, and fat—as well as water. *Obesity* refers specifically to having excess body fat. One can be overweight without being obese. For example, a bodybuilder who has a lot of muscle tissue may be very heavy, but not obese. Most people who are overweight are also obese. Obesity is one of those words that has one meaning to the layperson, and a more precise meaning to the medical world. To most people, to be obese means to be very overweight. To doctors and scientists, a person can be considered obese even if he or she isn't particularly overweight.

Three Ways to Measure Being Overweight

Measuring a person's body fat isn't easy, so doctors often rely on other means to diagnose obesity. Two widely used measurements are weight-for-height tables and body mass index (BMI). Both have their limitations, but both are good guides for you. And there is always what is known as the belt method.

WEIGHT-FOR-HEIGHT

You're probably familiar with weight-for-height tables that have a range of acceptable weights for your height. Many versions are printed in books and brochures. Some tables take a person's frame size, age, and sex into account; others do not. One of the problems of a weight-for-height table is that it does not distinguish between excess fat and good muscle. Some charts show that getting heavier and heavier as you age is normal. I don't agree. Many of my patients remain in good health because they remain fairly close to what they weighed in their early thirties. Check your weight and size using the charts below.

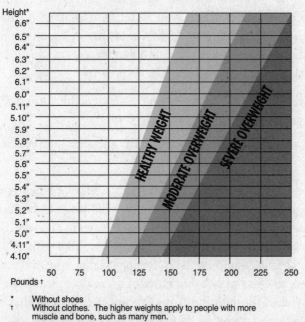

WEIGHT-FOR-HEIGHT CHART

* Without shoes
† Without clothes. The higher weights apply to people with more muscle and bone, such as many men.

Source: Report of the Dietary Guidelines Advisory Committee on the Dietary Guidelines for Americans, 1995, pages 23-24.

BODY MASS INDEX (BMI)

Body mass index, or BMI, a new term, is the measurement of choice for many researchers studying obesity. BMI uses a mathematical formula based on both a person's height and weight. BMI equals a person's weight divided by height. The table opposite has been modified and the math has been done for you. The BMI measurement poses some of the same problems as the weight-for-height tables. Doctors don't agree on the cutoff points for "healthy" versus "unhealthy" BMI ranges. The BMI also does not provide information on the percentage of body fat. However, it is a useful guideline.

THE BELT METHOD

If you're a woman and your waist measures more than 35 inches, or if you're a man and your waist measures more than 40 inches, you are more likely to develop high blood pressure and other health problems. Talk to your doctor.

Pears and Apples

The areas of your body where your fat tends to accumulate may be just as important as how much you weigh. A study in the *International Journal of Obesity* about a dozen years ago found that there were two distinct types of stored fat:

Fat carried below the waist, in thighs, hips, and buttocks, is called the "pear" shape.

Fat carried around and above the waist and abdomen is called the "apple" shape.

Doctors have developed a simple way to measure whether someone is an apple or a pear. The measurement is called waist-to-hip ratio. To find out someone's waist-to-hip ratio, measure the waist at its narrowest point, then measure the hips at the widest point. A woman with a 35-inch waist and 46-inch hips would do the following calculation: 35 divided by 46 = 0.76. Women with waist-to-hip ratios of more than .8, or men with waist-to-hip ratios of more than 1.0, are "apples." They are at increased health risk due to fat distribution.

Although many obesity experts say the jury is still out, above-the-waist

BODY WEIGHT IN POUNDS ACCORDING TO HEIGHT AND BODY MASS INDEX

Each entry gives the body weight in pounds (lbs) for a person of a given height and body mass index. Pounds have been rounded off. To use the table, find the appropriate height in the left-hand column. Move across the row to a given weight. The number at the top of the column is the body mass index for the height and weight. A BMI of more than 30 is usually considered a sign of obesity.

	BODY MASS INDEX (KG/M)													
	19	20	21	22	23	24	25	26	27	28	29	30	35	40
HT. (IN)	BODY WEIGHT (LBS)													
58	91	96	100	105	110	115	119	124	129	134	138	143	167	191
59	94	99	104	109	114	119	124	128	133	138	143	148	173	198
60	97	102	107	112	118	123	128	133	138	143	148	153	179	204
61	100	106	111	116	122	127	132	137	143	148	153	158	185	211
62	104	109	115	120	126	131	136	142	147	153	158	164	191	218
63	107	113	118	124	130	135	141	146	152	158	163	169	197	225
64	110	116	122	128	134	140	145	151	157	163	169	174	204	232
65	114	120	126	132	138	144	150	156	162	168	174	180	210	240
66	118	124	130	136	142	148	155	161	167	173	179	186	216	247
67	121	127	134	140	146	153	159	166	172	178	185	191	223	255
68	125	131	138	144	151	158	164	171	177	184	190	197	230	262
69	128	135	142	149	155	162	169	176	182	189	196	203	236	270
70	132	139	146	153	160	167	174	181	188	195	202	207	243	278
71	136	143	150	157	165	172	179	186	193	200	208	215	250	286
72	140	147	154	162	169	177	184	191	199	206	213	221	258	294
73	144	151	159	166	174	182	189	197	204	212	219	227	265	302
74	148	155	163	171	179	186	194	202	210	218	225	233	272	311
75	152	160	168	176	184	192	200	208	216	224	232	240	279	319
76	156	164	172	180	189	197	205	213	221	230	238	246	287	328

Source: Adapted with permission from G.A. Bray and D.S. Gray, "Obesity. Part 1. Pathogenesis." West J. Med. 1988;149:429–41.

fat could prove to be a risk factor for high cholesterol or hypertension. On the other hand, while fat thighs may be displeasing, from a medical standpoint they may not be as bad as a fat tummy.

GENDER AND BODY FAT

During the past decade there has been a great deal of research on the distribution of fat in the human body. It is likely that a number of genetic mechanisms influence weight, among them genes that dictate how you convert fat into energy. One study points to an enzyme produced by fat cells to help store calories as fat; if too much of this enzyme is produced, the body will be especially efficient at storing calories.

These enzymes are partly controlled by reproductive hormones (estrogen in women, testosterone in men), so gender differences in the activity of the enzyme are also a factor in obesity. In women, fat cells in the hips, thighs, and breasts secrete the enzyme. In men, the enzyme is produced by fat cells in the midriff region. Fat cells in the abdominal area release their contents for quick energy, while fat in the thighs and buttocks is used for long-term energy storage. So, a man can often pare his paunch more readily than a woman can shed fat from her thighs.

Why Should You Care?

Now that you've checked the charts and measured your waist, you know if you need to lose weight. Could conquering your obesity lower your blood pressure? Yes. Obesity is a known risk factor for several chronic diseases: diabetes, stroke, and even some forms of cancer, as well as high blood pressure.

Does obesity cause hypertension? While there is no clear evidence that it does, common sense and statistics suggest that anyone suffering from hypertension, or anyone who has a family potential for hypertension, would be smart to keep his or her weight down. Many experts think it is important for everyone.

Hypertension affects your vascular system. When you are overweight, you put an additional strain on your vascular system, because your body needs a greater blood supply to maintain it. You need increased blood flow to meet its metabolic needs. If you lose weight, you reduce the need for increased vascular function and heart action. For that reason alone, it makes sense to try to keep your weight within the healthy range.

Another way of understanding the dangers of being overweight is to consider what would happen if you placed a fifteen-pound weight on your back and kept it there for the entire day. You would find that you needed more energy to get about. Your heart would have to work harder to overcome this extra strain. Being overweight has the same effect.

Weight gain—whether added over a long period of time or piled on in just a few months—causes obesity. A gain in weight occurs when a person's caloric intake exceeds the amount of energy burned. What causes this imbalance between consuming and burning calories varies. The evidence suggests that obesity has many causes. Genetic, environmental, psychological, and other factors may all be involved.

Heredity vs. Conditioned Response

Is being fat hereditary? When we look at overweight fathers and sons or mothers and daughters who are identical in size and shape, it seems likely. Examples of this kind of obesity can be found in several generations of some families. This points to genetic predisposition. Studies have shown that in families where both parents are of normal weight, only 9 percent of the children are obese. On the other hand, when one parent is overweight, 40 percent of the children are obese, and when both parents are overweight, 80 percent of the children are obese.

Certainly, genes are a factor in being overweight, but many experts believe heredity affects only a small portion of vast numbers of people in America who are overweight. For instance, in one study of adults who were adopted as children, researchers found that the adult weight was very close to that of their biological parents, suggesting that being overweight is related to genetics.

It is therefore hard to say whether being overweight is the result of heredity or whether parents who eat too much teach their children to overeat, whereas thin parents set a different example for their children, who also stay thin. Certainly the kinds of diets that children are raised on, and learn to like, affect their ultimate body weight and structure. But you can take heart (figuratively and literally): no matter how your genes predispose your body to gain weight, you *can* manage to lose weight and keep it off.

LIFESTYLE FACTORS

Although genes are an important factor, environment plays a significant part in weight gain and weight loss. Your diet and activity can make a difference. Americans tend to eat large portions of high-fat foods. Those foods often have strong flavors, what food technologists call "mouth appeal." Many people choose their food based on its convenience, not its nutritional value, and this can put on unwanted pounds.

Since we cannot select our parents, but we can change what we eat, to lose weight we should:

* Choose nutritious meals that are low in fat.
* Recognize tempting cues such as the smells of certain foods. These cues make you want to eat when you're not hungry.
* Move more, do small active things—reach, bend, walk. Become more physically active.
* Monitor emotional states.

Your mind and emotions also affect your eating habits. In the movies and in the theater, when people are upset, they don't eat. In real life, many people respond to boredom, sadness, anger, or depression by eating. Happy social events are also food-centered; weddings, banquets, and celebrations often involve large elaborate meals.

Binge eating affects about one in every three people who are seriously overweight. Those with the most severe binge problems are considered to have an eating disorder, and these people may have more difficulty than others when they attempt to lose weight and keep it off.

HEALTH FACTORS

Other causes of obesity may include a thyroid imbalance, Cushing's syndrome (caused by an adrenal or pituitary dysfunction), and certain neurologic problems. Some drugs may cause weight gain. Remember: Before attempting any weight loss, it is important to discuss your plans with your physician.

Who Should Lose Weight?

Anyone who is 20 percent or more overweight can enjoy substantial health benefits from weight loss. Many experts believe that if you are above your recommended weight, if you have any of the risk factors I've listed below, you should consider a weight loss program.

◆ Family history of chronic illness, such as heart disease or diabetes.

◆ Preexisting medical condition, such as high blood pressure, high choles- terol levels, or high blood sugar levels.

◆ An apple-shaped body with most of your weight at the waist and above. This shape puts you at greater risk of heart disease, diabetes, or cancer than those who are pear-shaped.

◆ Gender is a factor; men who have a higher muscle weight in their body use about 10 percent more calories than women. If you have a low muscle-to-fat ratio, consider weight loss. As you get older, your percent- age of muscle tends to drop; as a result, your body fat burns more slowly. Together, these changes can put on the pounds.

A series of long-term studies conducted at the Gerontology Research Center in Baltimore, Maryland, found that people in their sixties who are somewhat overweight, but not obese, had a better chance of living to their eighties and nineties than those who are normal weight or under. Notwith- standing that news, even a small weight loss—ten or twenty pounds—can lower your blood pressure and cholesterol levels.

Obesity Risk Factors

Losing weight isn't just about looking better and finding new clothes easily and feeling more confident when you meet people. Fat is a health hazard. Someone who is 40 percent overweight is twice as likely to die prematurely than a person of average weight. The annual number of deaths attributed to poor diet and inactivity is a staggering 300,000.

Hypertension seldom has symptoms, but obesity always does. We can see the symptoms in our mirrors. Here are some diseases correlated with obesity:

◆ Non-insulin-dependent diabetes mellitus: Nearly 80 percent of patients are obese.

◆ Gallbladder disease: The incidence of gallstones soars with a BMI (body mass index) over 29.

◆ Heart disease: Nearly 70 percent of cases of cardiovascular disease are related to obesity.

- Stroke: this is a high risk factor for obese people.

- Breast and colon cancer: Almost half of breast cancer cases are diagnosed among obese women. Obese women are more likely than non-obese women to die from cervical and ovarian cancers. An estimated 42 percent of colon cancer cases are diagnosed among the obese.

- Osteoarthritis: In this disease, the joints, under pressure of excess weight, deteriorate.

- Gout: Affecting the joints, the disease is more common in overweight people. (Note: Over the short term, some diets may lead to an attack of gout in people who have high levels of uric acid or who have had gout. Check with your doctor before trying to lose weight.)

- Respiratory problems: One example is sleep apnea, when breathing is stopped for a time during sleep.

Obesity Takes a Psychological and Social Toll

One of the most painful aspects of obesity may be the emotional suffering it causes. American society places a high value on physical appearance. People often equate attractiveness with slimness. This is especially true for women, but in recent years children and young men are also being pressured to remain slim. The messages, intended or not, make overweight people feel unattractive.

Many people assume that obese people are gluttonous, lazy, or both. However, more and more evidence contradicts this assumption. Obese people often face prejudice or discrimination in many aspects of life. A recent study of women workers in corporations showed that obese women are paid less than their slim sisters and are often ignored at meetings. Feelings of rejection, shame, or depression are common in obese people of both sexes.

Treatments for Obesity

Treatment options for obesity are touted on television and in magazines; books are written on how to lose weight; celebrities discuss their own weight-loss techniques. The methods that you select and that work for you are individual. Slow and steady weight loss of about one half to one pound a week is considered the safest way to lose weight—and to keep that weight off. Very rapid weight loss can cause you to lose muscle rather than fat. The treatments that have been found most successful—and that have lowered high blood pressure—include combinations of diet, exercise, and behavior modification.

If you're not overweight but hypertension runs in your family, or you have other hypertension risk factors, it is important that you try to keep your weight down. There are many sections in this book that will give you easy-to-follow methods on how to improve your diet.

TOM AND JANE LOSE TO GAIN

Tom, at age 30, has had essential hypertension. His problem was compounded by his weighing 240 pounds, far too much for his five-foot-eleven frame. Tom took two antihypertensive pills a day to keep his blood pressure down. Finally, because of side effects—from the antihypertensives, his hypertension itself, and the weight he was carrying around—he went on a diet. As soon as he started to lose weight, Tom's blood pressure went down. By the time he weighed 180 pounds, his pressure was normal *without medication.*

Jane had a different experience. Jane weighed 110 pounds and was about five feet three inches tall, with normal blood pressure. Then her career seemed to take off. Jane became an office supervisor and her weight started to climb along with her blood pressure. Over the next five years, Jane's weight rose to 150 pounds, her blood pressure to 150/95. I put Jane on a strict weight-reduction program primarily to control her seriously elevated pressure. As Jane lost weight, her blood pressure came down too. Each time her weight went up, however, her blood pressure measurements reflected the change and went back up.

For both Tom and Jane, as for so many people, body weight and hypertension obviously were related. Once Jane realized this fact, she was motivated to get back to her previously normal weight and stay there.

Are you thinking, "Easier said than done"? The past decade has brought great advances in understanding obesity. Fighting obesity—without drugs—can change your life and increase your feeling of self-control and self-esteem. It can also lower your blood pressure. And it just might save your life.

CHAPTER 9

Are You Really Hungry?

If you are appreciably heavier than the recommended weight for your age, height, and sex—it is time for a change. Don't be fooled into thinking that weight means little in your particular case because you feel just fine. Remember that you can feel great and have no obvious symptoms, yet still have high blood pressure.

Weight control is key to hypertension control. Science backs up what I'm saying, and so does my personal experience with hypertensive patients.

What I Did for Myself

We all know the old chestnut "Physician heal thyself." As a physician, I've been reminded of this more than once. I try to keep my own waistline as slim as it was several decades ago, which isn't always easy. But I did get some help a few years ago when I shared an office with a psychiatrist. She kept our small office refrigerator filled with packages of carrots and celery sticks, apples, and melons cut into bite-size pieces. She insisted that when I craved a snack, I would soon become accustomed to eating these foods rather than cookies, cake, or ice cream—and she was right! After gradually acquiring a taste for foods that were good for me, I came to like them and I learned that I could survive on a diet both physically and emotionally rewarding.

My breakfast is usually half a grapefruit (the entire grapefruit if I am hungry) or any other fresh fruit. Sometimes I enjoy half a piece of whole wheat toast, or half a bagel. Rather than jelly, I use prune butter or apple butter. I often drink two cups of coffee, both with skim milk.

Ignorance Is Not Bliss

Most women at her age would have retired, but at 66, Ida had a working active busy life. Standing five feet five inches tall, Ida never weighed more than 135 pounds, until she was in her mid-fifties. However, like many post-menopausal women she began to gain, and by her sixties, Ida weighed 170 pounds.

Ida felt great and had more energy than her 32-year-old daughter. So why bother seeing a doctor for a checkup? Then, luckily as it turned out, Ida came down with flu. (I don't think she bothered with flu shots, either.) When her fever reached 103°, Ida took a cab to her physician's office. During a routine office examination and blood pressure check, her high blood pressure was discovered.

Ida was immediately placed on antihypertensive medication and put on a weight loss diet. As her weight came down and her pressure fell, she needed fewer and fewer antihypertensive medications. In fact, as long as she adhered to her diet and watched her intake of salt, Ida controlled her hypertension with minimal medication.

Lunch is usually an apple. If I go out to lunch, I order a small salad and use lemon as a dressing. If I'm still hungry I have another small fruit. My change from a standard hamburger lunch to salad or a fresh fruit could be considered a minor miracle.

For dinner, I start with a large vegetable salad. I find that this fills me up so well that I can limit the calories in any main course. For dessert, my best bets are a simple fruit salad or fresh fruit. I've learned to enjoy only the simplest of foods; no heavy sauces for me. The diet has not always been easy, but after I became accustomed to it, I never felt deprived. It has been worth it for my health.

Here are some tips I've learned: I spend time preparing the meal. I cut salad greens and raw vegetables into small pieces and I use bright red tomatoes or red bell peppers for a garnish so that the salad looks attractive. I use no salt, but I use my elegant pepper mill freely. Drinking water while eating is not ideal, since it dilutes the gastric enzymes needed for digestion, so I drink a glass of water one half an hour before the meal. This allows time for my stomach to tell my brain that I'm not empty.

Understanding Why You Eat (When You're Not Hungry)

So why do people overeat when they know it's bad for them? I think it works like this: Eating represents many things to many people, and people eat for many reasons other than simple hunger. If you can understand *why* you eat too much you can prepare a strategy to overcome that problem. Do any of these reasons for eating too much or too often sound familiar?

- I eat because the food is too appealing to avoid.
- I eat because I love to eat.
- I eat because I feel I mustn't waste food—I clean up my plate.
- I eat when I'm bored.
- I eat when I'm depressed (or angry, nervous, upset, tired).
- I eat when I'm relaxed and happy and feel like celebrating.

The list is really endless, but to recognize the cause of your problem is the first step to lower weight and blood pressure. It isn't always easy at first, but it becomes a pleasant part of your lifestyle as time goes by.

RECOGNIZING REAL HUNGER

True hunger is a physiological reaction to the need for food. The brain feels hunger long before the stomach. You may feel no stomach discomfort, but hunger can manifest itself as a lack of energy or a headache. The body—especially the brain—needs blood sugar to function, and when blood

---

Chew Away the Fat?

Lose weight by chewing gum? According to a December 1999 *New York Times* article, chewing sugarless gum for twelve minutes at the rate of 100 chews a minute might help people lose up to eleven pounds in a year. However, Dr. James Levine of the Mayo Clinic doesn't advocate this form of "exercise." He said, "People who really needed to lose weight would be better off exercising more and watching what they eat." But since doing his experiment, Levine says he chews gum all the time. Personally, I've found that keeping my mouth shut when confronted with high-calorie foods is better than chewing.

Do You Live "Hand to Mouth"?

Before you eat a large-size anything . . . think:

* What am I really craving?
* Am I really hungry or do I want something else?
* What is the reason I want to eat?

---

sugar levels are decreased, there is a desire for food. There are other, as yet not understood, factors that affect the hunger center which exists in the pea-sized master gland in the middle of the brain called the hypothalamus. The sensation of hunger, from stomach pangs to intestinal rumbles, arises from this central control. Appetite is a psychological response. Emotions, habits, and the memory of how good some foods taste all stir appetite.

When we have eaten enough, we have a sense of satiation, and this should be the signal to stop eating. Humans have the unfortunate ability to override this feeling. For example, you can eat ice cream even after you have consumed a large meal. You can eat when you wish, not just when your body requires nourishment. You should learn to control your appetite by recognizing those internal signals that the body produces in response to a true need for food. Learn to distinguish between true hunger and the desire to simply keep on eating. Before you eat, ask yourself if you are hungry or if you are responding to other stimuli. Eat only when you are hungry and only the amount needed to satisfy your feelings of hunger. Tip: One of my patients told me that when she feels hungry but isn't *really* hungry, she brushes her teeth. It not only seems to provide some sort of oral stimulation, but it keeps her teeth clean and shiny.

Scientific knowledge about what causes the feeling of satiation is less advanced than an understanding of what causes hunger. When science develops a clearer explanation of satiation, it will be possible to produce this response, which in turn will help people lose weight.

Learned Habits

If you answer yes, agreeing that the following food cues make you hungry, you are responding to food cues and not true hunger. Try to avoid these trigger situations.

- Seeing someone eating a big, salty pretzel or a cookie
- Popcorn fragrance in a movie theater
- Smelling baked foods such as fresh bread or cookies
- Just thinking of spicy or garlic-flavored foods such as hot dogs
- When in a restaurant, seeing wonderful large orders carried by the servers

A Lifetime of Consequences

There are many reasons why overfeeding a child often results in an obese adult. Early in childhood and during adolescence, food intake determines the number of fat cells developed in the body for the remainder of your life.

A child who is overfed will develop a large number of fat cells. Without overfeeding, a child's body will produce only the number of fat cells needed for his or her size. Thus, parents should also be careful not to make food a reward. Children rewarded with cakes, candy, and ice cream may grow into adults who reward themselves with the same treats! This is a conditioned response. You may have gotten off to the wrong start as child, but it isn't too late to make adjustments in your present eating habits.

Rocky Road Ice Cream

A couple who had been married for a year are an example of learned behavior. I suggested that the wife, who weighed 190 pounds and was having some medical problems, should reduce her weight. The young wife said, "I can't lose weight because my husband brings ice cream home and gets me to eat it with him." He agreed, saying, "I can't help it. I love ice cream and I was unable to have it when I was young, so I really enjoy it now." The couple had "learned" that ice cream tastes wonderful, and just couldn't resist the pleasure of eating it. Note: This couple are expecting a child. Unless something changes, the child will be part of a home of overeaters.

The Plus Side of Weight Management

Developing a plan to keep your weight and your blood pressure down has many bonuses. You are in control of what you put in your mouth. You can keep your calorie intake at the level you want, and when you meet your weight goal, you can enjoy the feeling of self-control it gives you. Once you've reached your desired weight, don't let go. Continue all the plans and strategies that worked, for they can help you maintain your desired weight. Reward yourself, not with a forbidden food, but with a smaller belt size.

CHAPTER 10

Eat Right/Feel Right

Have you decided to control your HBP by reducing your weight and your belt size? If you have, good! There are some facts you should know before you start a weight loss plan. Importantly, you should understand that obesity is a condition, not a moral failing.

As an October 8, 1999, *New York Times* article stated: "To link dieting success or failure with willpower is to ignore the complex interaction of brain chemicals, behavior conditioning, hormones, heredity, and the powerful influence of habits. Telling an overweight person to use willpower is like telling a clinically depressed person to 'snap out of it.'" The article quotes many weight loss researchers in debunking the myth that all you need is willpower.

It isn't easy. Overweight people must manage their lives to avoid confronting situations that make willpower an issue.

How We Lose Weight

Your body weight is controlled by the number of calories you eat and the number of calories you use each day. So, to lose weight, you need to take in fewer calories than you use. A calorie is a measure of energy. In medicine and nutrition, calories indicate the energy content of foods and the energy used to perform all of our activities. The energy needed varies depending on age, sex, and physical activity. Most nutritionists think that we need to run a deficit of 3,500 calories to lose one pound. Even a deficit of 100 or 200 calories a day will add up, day after day, and at the end of a week, you will

> ## Convenience Makes You Fat
>
> Fifty-five percent of adult Americans are now overweight, up from 46 percent ten years ago. Convenience may be a contributing factor. The *International Journal of Obesity* estimates that with the advent of remote controls, elevators, escalators, dishwashers, and the Internet, average energy expenditures have dropped 800 calories a day in the past thirty years. For example, if you use the remote control instead of getting up to change channels, and shop on the Internet instead of going to the grocery store or mall once a week, you could gain almost forty pounds in a decade.

see a weight loss. Many experts recommend losing no more than a pound a week.

Weight Loss Products and Programs

There is no quick and easy way to lose weight. An estimated 50 million Americans go on a diet each year, and some of them lose weight. However, only about 5 percent actually keep the weight off. Unfortunately, most people find that as soon as their weight goes back up, their blood pressure also rises.

Dieting to reduce weight isn't fast or easy. The problems are compounded by the need to reduce sodium, and many people turn to weight loss products. The weight loss business is a booming industry full of hopes and promises. But you should beware of the scams out there. Here are the general points to keep in mind:

- Any claims that you can lose weight effortlessly are false. The only proven way to lose weight is either to reduce the number of calories you eat or to increase the number of calories expended.
- Very low-calorie diets are not without risk, and require medical supervision.
- Fad diets rarely have any permanent effect. So-called crash diets often are followed by quick gain or rebound weight gains, making the next dieting attempt even more difficult.

Fasting—not eating at all—doesn't work. Your body needs certain nutrients to keep you thinking and moving, and to fuel your body systems.

Too Good to Be True

It is important for consumers to be wary of claims that sound too good to be true. When it comes to weight loss, be skeptical of claims containing words and phrases such as:

easily	breakthrough secret
effortless	ancient
miraculously	exclusive
magical	

To report fraudulent weight loss product claims, contact your state attorney general, local consumer protection office, or Better Business Bureau. Fraudulent claims are dishonest and some are dangerous.

The first step to reduce your weight is to reduce your food intake by half. For example, if you are accustomed to eating a sandwich at lunch—eat only half. This may seem simplistic, but I've found it effective. Another plus is that reducing the volume of what you eat makes changing to a nutritionally sound diet easier.

Some people count calories; others find calorie counting confusing and time-consuming. If you do keep a record of what you eat, it will help you replace high-calorie foods with lower calorie foods. The challenge is using your ingenuity to get the most usable nutrition in foods with the fewest calories.

Perilous Pills

In 1992, the Weight Loss Practices Survey, sponsored by the Federal Drug Administration (FDA) and the National Heart, Lung, and Blood Institute, found that many women and some men who were trying to lose weight used diet pills to suppress their appetite. Over-the-counter weight control drugs are primarily those containing the active ingredient phenylpropanolamine (PPA). Because of a number of problems, PPA was taken from the market in the summer of 2000. If you have any medications that list PPA as an ingredient, it is best to throw that medication away.

The FDA has approved several prescription drugs for treating obesity. Studies show that for people on calorie-restricted diets, those who took the drugs lost more weight on average than those who took a placebo (a "dummy" medication that contains no real medicine). But the amount of weight lost varied and tended to be just a fraction of a pound each week.

The biggest drawback to pills, as far as I'm concerned, is that drugs of any kind can't help in learning to eat a new way or in changing lifestyle habits. To achieve long-term weight loss and to enjoy the improved self-esteem that comes with taking charge of your life, finding a diet you can live with and increasing your physical activity is the right way to go.

Just How Many Calories Do You Need?

How much food you should consume depends on many factors: your height, your size, your age, your sex, and your activities. People come in all sizes and shapes, and some people gain and lose weight more easily than others.

Generally, young people need 2,400 to 3,000 calories per day; but most of us with high blood pressure are older and less active than these sample young adults. Sedentary workers—those who sit in a car or in front of a computer—just don't require as many calories as those who are farmers, fishermen, dancers, athletes, or even physicians. Weight-reduction diets can range from 1,000 to 2,200 calories a day. A deficit of about 500 calories a day will result in losing about one pound a week. The main idea is to take in fewer calories each day than your body normally needs for maintenance. This sort of diet should produce a slow, constant weight loss.

Such a diet allows your body to adjust to the new level of calories. A 2,000-calorie maintenance diet is usually at the right level for someone who is only moderately active. If you find it is too high or too low, you can adjust your intake. The goal is to become accustomed to eating the right foods in the right proportions.

Welcome to DASH

First published in 1998 and reprinted in 1999, DASH (Dietary Approaches to Stop Hypertension) was a research study designed to test the effect of dietary patterns on blood pressure. The study found that a diet reduced in

Where Does DASH Come From?

The DASH diet developed from a study that was sponsored by the National Heart, Lung, and Blood Institute and was conducted at four medical sites: Brigham and Woman's Hospital, Boston, Massachusetts; Duke University Medical Center, Durham, North Carolina; Johns Hopkins University, Baltimore, Maryland; and Pennington Biomedical Research Center, Louisiana State University, Baton Rouge, Louisiana. There was also a central coordinating site at Kaiser Permanente Center for Health Research in Portland, Oregon.

total and saturated fat but rich in fruits, vegetables, and low-fat dairy foods can lower blood pressure as much as an antihypertensive medication. (Alert: This *doesn't* mean that you can stop taking prescribed medication without checking with your physician.) The development of DASH is important for everyone with HBP.

DASH researchers compared three eating plans, each at about 3,000 calories, the average amount consumed by Americans. The first was a plan similar to the way many Americans actually eat, featuring many fatty foods. The second was higher than average in fruits and vegetables. The third was a combination plan—the DASH diet—lower in all fats and cholesterol, yet very rich in fruits, vegetables, and low-fat dairy foods.

Results showed that both the fruit-vegetable and combination plans (plans 2 and 3) reduce blood pressure. However, the combination plan (3) had the greatest effect. The DASH eating plan reduced blood pressure by an average of 6 mm Hg for systolic pressure and 3 mm Hg diastolic pressure. It worked even better for those with very high blood pressure; the systolic dropped an average of about 11 mm Hg and the diastolic about 6 mm Hg. Best of all, the reductions came fast—within two weeks of starting the eating plan. The DASH plan may have more servings of fruits, vegetables, and grains than you are used to. To avoid bloating from this high-fiber plan, increase your servings of fruits, grains, and vegetables very gradually. (See Chapter 13 for more on the importance of fiber.)

Appendix 2 (pages 317–24) is a one-week plan for the DASH diet. I like this diet because it is doable. The recipes for the starred dishes can be found in the recipes section, Chapter 33. I especially like including snacks; having an afternoon snack makes me feel as if I'm really not dieting at all.

DASH Nutrients

The DASH diet is rich in nutrients; if you eat about 2,000 calories a day on the plan, you will be getting:

4,500 milligrams potassium

500 milligrams magnesium

1,240 milligrams calcium

The DASH diet provides about two or three times the amounts of these minerals most Americans get.

GETTING STARTED

How can you get started on DASH? It's easy! The DASH plan requires no special foods and has no hard-to-follow recipes with exotic ingredients. One way to begin is by seeing how DASH compares with your current food habits. Keep a record of what you eat for one to two days and see how your diet compares with the DASH plan. This will help you see what you need to change.

Remember that some days you may eat more than what's recommended from one food group and less of another. But don't worry. Just be sure that the average of several days or weeks comes close to what's recommended. Note: It is important for you to continue monitoring your blood pressure and taking any medication your doctor has prescribed. Do not stop or change your HBP therapy without the approval of your doctor.

Change gradually:

- Eat one or two vegetables a day, add another serving at lunch or dinner. Or, if you don't eat fruit now, add a fresh fruit at breakfast.
- Use only half the butter and salad dressing you do now.
- Try low-fat or fat-free condiments, such as fat-free salad dressings.
- Gradually increase dairy products to three servings a day, using low-fat or skim milk dairy products.
- Cut down on meat. Treat meat as one ingredient in a meal—not the focus. Eat vegetables with meat, not meat with vegetables. Buy less meat. If it's not there, you won't eat it. Limit meat to 6 ounces a day (two small

servings, each no larger than a deck of cards). Cut back gradually on meat consumption.

- Include two or more vegetarian-style meals each week. Tip: Mushroom-based dishes can mimic the texture and taste of meat. Tofu is also a good meat substitute, and it is high in calcium. A little meat mixed with grains and beans is as filling as a meat dish.

- Use fruits or low-fat foods as desserts. Use fresh or frozen fruits for special treats. Try fruits with raisins, low-fat graham crackers, low-fat and fat-free yogurt and frozen yogurt.

New Ways of Eating

The DASH eating plan is meant for people with elevated blood pressure. It is also a heart-happy plan that you can share with your family. The DASH plan is a new way of eating—for a lifetime. If you slip and don't follow the eating plan once or even for a few days, don't get discouraged. Everyone slips—especially when learning something new. Remember that changing your lifestyle is a long-term process. Don't let a few slips keep you from reaching your health goals. Just get back on track.

One of the best ways of keeping on track is finding out why you slipped: Was it a party? Was there an unusual stress in your life? Were you trying to change too much about your life too fast? Were you watching television? Were you feeling tired? When you pinpoint the situations that are most likely to make you slip, you can figure out ways of avoiding temptation. Keep a DASH snack at the ready for those times. Some people find that raw baby carrots and celery sticks provide lots of "bite" appeal, and are filling as well.

CHAPTER 11

The Rice Diet and Other Diet Choices

I like rice. Our family eats rice at least twice a week, and has come up with some inventive ways of combining rice with seasonings to make it taste sweet, savory, or spicy. Best of all, rice is a wonderful food for anyone who is concerned about high blood pressure.

Dr. Kempner's Discovery: The Rice Diet

About fifty years ago a major advance in understanding the relationship between diet and the treatment of hypertension was made by Dr. Walter Kempner of Duke University. He was responsible for what has come to be known as the rice diet. Here is how it happened: A thirty-three-year-old woman suffering from severe kidney disease was told to remain on a diet of plain unsalted rice for two weeks and then to return for further evaluation. However, the woman did not return for two months.

When Kempner finally examined her, he found a remarkable difference: Her blood pressure had come down, and her electrocardiogram had improved, as had the serious aspects of her kidney disease. Seeing this marked change, Kempner intuitively realized long-term dietary treatment could be helpful, while short-term diet was too brief to produce positive results. Kempner's findings were amazing. In almost two thirds of his patients who adopted a similar rice diet, blood pressure decreased, kidney function improved, and cardiac muscle was strengthened.

This marked the first use of low-salt diets to treat patients with high blood pressure. In fact it was the only successful treatment before the

Varieties of Rice

Arborio: A short-grained rice that becomes creamy when cooked.

Basmati: A long-grained, nutty-flavored rice; it has the aroma of popcorn when cooking.

Brown rice: A long-cooking, nutty flavored rice with high food value.

Converted rice: Hulled under moist conditions, steamed, and dried so that all the nutrients are incorporated back into the grain. The texture is pasty.

Dehydrated precooked rice (Instant or Minute Rice): Packaged flavored rice may be high in sodium; the outside seems fluffy, but the center may remain raw.

White rice: The outer covering has been removed by polishing. The same process takes away the B vitamins. Long-grain white rice is the most popular in the United States.

Wild rice: Not really a rice, but a seed from a grass that grows wild along the edges of lakes in Minnesota, Wisconsin, and southern Canada. It is expensive, dark in color, and has a strong, unique flavor. It is best mixed with other rices.

present-day antihypertensive medications. Today, low-salt diets continue to be an important part of high blood pressure treatment.

DRAWBACKS TO THE RICE DIET

Given the success of the rice diet, what prevents its widespread use? If it was so good, why isn't every hypertensive on a rice diet? Unfortunately, the rice diet is difficult to follow. The present rice diet consists of rice, fruit, vinegar and no salt, and drinking between twenty-four and forty ounces of liquid daily. The rice diet has twice as much carbohydrate as is in the average American's diet, one fourth as much protein, and less than one twentieth the amount of fat. The rice diet does not provide many of the nutrients that the human body needs. Another hurdle blocking the universal use of the rice diet is its monotony—eating plain rice daily is not very exciting.

The rice diet also requires days of preliminary diagnostic observation before a person starts the program, and months of treatment. During this time, patients must consume only special meals. The rice diet can be so expensive and time-consuming that some hypertension patients need a support group to stay on it.

However, when you weigh all these drawbacks against the possibility of high blood pressure leading to stroke, heart attack, heart failure, and hypertension-induced sexual dysfunction such as impotence in the male, the diet may not be so hard to accept after all. The diet is not for all hypertensives.

WHY RICE?

When Dr. Kempner chose rice as the staple of the diet, it was not a purely fortuitous decision. Rice is good food for hypertensives. It is salt- and cholesterol-free, low in calories, high in bulk, and easy to prepare.

Furthermore, rice is not a newcomer to the pages of medical history. As far back as 1897, it was noted that poultry fed on polished rice developed a disease of the nervous system. When chickens ate the part of the rice discarded during polishing, the symptoms of the disease abated. The missing essential ingredient was found to be vitamin B_1, or thiamine.

Since most Americans prefer white rice, methods have been developed whereby rice can be parboiled—or converted—before milling to preserve some of its nutritional value. In this process, the unmilled rice is soaked

Low Count

The trade-off in nutritive content is balanced by a low sodium content and a low fat content. (The values given here are for rice cooked in water to which no salt has been added.) Here are some nutrition facts about rice:

1 ounce of brown rice has 3 mg of sodium

1 ounce of converted rice has 6 mg of sodium

1 ounce of white rice has less than 1 mg of sodium

1 cup of cooked brown rice has 200 calories

1 cup of cooked converted rice has 188 calories

1 cup of cooked white rice has 184 calories

in water just under the boiling point and then steamed under pressure. This pressure forces some of the nutritional material from the bran layer into the inner rice grain. Converted (parboiled) rice has greater nutritional value than does ordinary white rice.

SODIUM AND CALORIE CONTENT OF RICE

Rice has a long history and has been cultivated in almost every area of the world; it is probably consumed by more people than any other grain. Rice supplies 55 percent of man's daily food requirements, and one pound of rice has four times the food energy of the same weight of potatoes.

Supermarkets offer a wide variety of rice products in addition to the three varieties of the grain itself. There are rice breakfast cereals, rice flours, and even rice wine. One particularly interesting rice product is the rice cake, which is a good replacement for junk food snacks. It comes in chewy four-inch wafers that are salt- and cholesterol-free and contain only 35 calories per wafer. Rice cakes have the advantage of being good for you while satisfying your hunger.

Middle Eastern Spiced Rice

SERVES 4

2 tablespoons olive oil

1 medium onion, chopped

½ cup chopped leftover raw vegetables (celery, tomatoes, carrots are fine)

½ cup mushrooms, sliced

½ cup green or red bell peppers, chopped

1 cup uncooked converted long-grain rice

2 cups water

⅛ teaspoon black pepper

1 teaspoon of your favorite spice

1 tablespoon nuts (almonds or walnut pieces)

Heat the oil in a deep skillet. Add the onions and vegetables; simmer until soft. Add rice and stir until the rice browns. Add the water, black pepper, and spice. Cover and cook about 22 minutes, or until rice is tender. Toss in nuts and serve.

Although Duke University's rice diet is effective, it's not more widely adopted because researchers continue to develop various medications that reduce blood pressure, regardless of diet. Moreover, drugs known as diuretic agents enable the kidneys to lose salt, duplicating the effects of a low-salt diet.

The rice diet is too rigorous an approach and too difficult to maintain for most people, but fortunately the choice is not just between medication and the rice diet. My patients have a great deal of success by simply eating more rice.

Other Diet Choices

If the DASH or rice diets don't appeal to you, you can devise your own eating program. We're all unique; what works for one person may spell failure and even weight gain for someone else. Over the years, my patients have come up with various methods and combinations of those methods that worked for them and were convenient for their lifestyle. Here are some of the dieting approaches they've told me about, and that I've tried. (Remember: The basic idea of all weight loss is to eat fewer calories than you usually eat and to stay as active as possible, increasing your activities if you can. This will maximize calorie burning.)

Fixed menu diets: This type of diet provides a list of all the foods you can eat. It is easy to follow because the foods are selected; you can eat only those food items on the list—no others. But such a diet is boring and has a built-in guilt factor that comes into play if you eat anything not listed. Another problem is that most of us eat away from home occasionally or often. Adhering to a specific list is burdensome and sometimes difficult or even impossible. In addition, you don't learn food selection skills.

Exchange diets: These programs have a set number of servings from each of several food groups. Within each group there can be an interchange of food items. For example, the starch category could include one slice of bread or about one-half cup of unsugared cereal—about the same nutritional value. With exchange diet programs there is some variety. You can modify the plan to accommodate impulse eating. They also allow you to eat out with a group of friends, and make transfers so that you eat what your friends or others will be eating. They also help you learn about food, calorie, and nutrition values and to make choices to suit your own taste.

Packaged meal diets: These programs require you to buy prepackaged meals. These meals may help people learn about appropriate portion size (smaller than you think). But the meals can be costly, and you don't learn how to select your own foods. (Also beware: Many packaged or convenience foods are high in sodium, which is used in preservatives and as a flavor-enhancer.)

Formula diets: These plans usually replace one or more meals with a liquid diet formula. (These are often advertised on television.) Formula diets are easy to use and do promote short-term weight loss, but most people regain the weight as soon as they make their own food choices. An apple or other fresh fruit, on the other hand, is a tried and true "packaged food" that also provides nutritional value and fiber.

Flexible diets: Some programs suggest counting only fat or only calories. This flexible approach works for some people and it teaches people to notice what they eat. But such a diet isn't really a total eating plan. The tendency is to cut the fat—but load up on the sugar. That does not lead to weight loss.

Questionable diets: You should avoid any diet that suggests you eat only a certain nutrient. One of the most deleterious aspects of single-food diets—including the rice diet—is that they are not balanced and may cause nutrient deficiencies. According to a diet exposé in a January 2000 article in the *New York Times,* you should not be impressed by testimonials of weight losses of dozens of pounds in just a short time. Weight experts say that no matter what diet you choose, you will feel great at first and then, as time wears on, hunger will come roaring back. This is especially true with one-food diets. If you're allowed to eat as much bacon as you want, you may think it's great. But what is it really doing to your body? This is true for every one-food diet, even the low-salt rice diet, which must be monitored closely by your physician.

Whether you use the DASH diet or count calories and nutrients yourself, choose an eating plan you can live with—for life! If you have high blood pressure, you will have to watch your diet throughout your life. (As most of us do anyway—especially since most people gain weight as they age.) Eating a healthful and nutritious diet to maintain your new weight, combined with regular physical activity, will prevent regaining weight.

Food Management Methods

Now that you know how many calories you need each day, I'd like to add some things you can do when trying to eliminate calorie- and salt-loaded foods from your life:

- Don't go shopping for food when you are hungry. I have made careful note of the food shopping I've done after lunch as opposed to the shopping I've done when I am hungry. Hungry people often buy foods they would not consider if they were full and satisfied. The safest way to shop is to make a list of those food items you need and include on that list only the foods in your diet plan—and go to the supermarket right after you've eaten. There are two bonuses in following this plan: You spend less on food and you throw away fewer food items.

- Don't shop every day. Shop as seldom as possible. Refrigerators with meat compartments and vegetable crispers are great for storage. However, many people who are binge eaters will find it best not to store large amounts of food.

- Do not buy items on impulse. Just because peach ice cream is on sale does not mean you must buy the gallon size and indulge yourself. And don't reach for that jar of pickles just because you saw that pickles ad on TV the night before. Stay with your predetermined diet plan. Have your list and adhere to it. Buy nothing else.

- Prepare in advance for the TV hunger rush—that sudden craving to eat something when you are watching television. Keep celery sticks, carrots, pineapple pieces, sunflower seeds, raisins, diet soda, and no-salt, no-butter popcorn on hand. Or make a bailout emergency list of your own to meet this problem.

- Do not keep salty, fatty, or calorie-rich snack foods at home. I find that if cookies or cakes that I like are easily available in the kitchen, the temptation is too great. If these foods are not available, I will happily eat an apple, a banana, or other fruit as a substitute. As a matter of fact, I have gotten so that I no longer enjoy candy as I did in the past—it tastes too sweet! Here's a trick for those of you with kids: Buy them cookies they like but you don't—that way you won't be tempted after they go to bed by that bag of cookies you know is in the cabinet.

- A food scale is an invaluable aid in controlling your food intake. Many foods can be eaten in small amounts, even though they are high in calories—if you limit the amount you eat. If you can safely have three ounces of an item, you can use the scale to measure the weight exactly.

- Be aware of what you are eating. Keep an accurate record of all you eat. In reviewing your daily intake of food, it sometimes comes as a shock to discover how much more you are eating than you thought, and how many more high-salt, high-fat foods than you thought.

- Weigh yourself, and cheer yourself on for your fortitude, as you record your successes. Don't be angry with yourself because of your failures. Being overly hard on yourself can discourage you and break your diet. If your weight starts to go back up, reduce your intake the next day to help balance the increase. Even if you do well dieting, there will be times when you go off your diet for one reason or another. Do not allow this slight deviation to be the end of your diet. On the contrary, use the deviation to help you get back to dieting with greater resolve. Use the scale to measure how well you are doing. After a while you won't even need the scale—just looking in the mirror will tell all. After a while you won't even have to look in the mirror—you'll become so attuned to your body that you'll know by how your body feels whether you're eating properly or not.

- When you have lost some weight and maintained the loss for a week or so, wear your belt on a tighter hole, or wear snug clothing. The smaller size is a great incentive to encourage you to stay at your new weight. As soon as the clothing starts to get a little tight, you know you should get down to some serious dieting again.

Eating Out

Americans enjoy eating out. We eat breakfast, lunch, and dinner away from home. Fast food restaurants send us off to a day's work or play, as do more formal cafés, delis, bistros, and other eateries. Some of us have to travel for business and so are often eating in restaurants. Choosing the food you eat out is just as important as shopping wisely for homemade meals.

Choose any restaurant you patronize carefully. Are there low-fat as well as low-sodium and high-fiber selections on the menu? Is there a salad bar? How are the meat, chicken, and fish dishes cooked? Can you have menu

> ### Chew on This
>
> Many people find that changing the way they chew food can help. If you chew food slowly, you will find you feel more satisfied with less food. Pause between bites. Allow a few seconds to pass before taking another bite and chewing it. You can increase your sense of satiation with less food simply by spending more time eating. Indeed, there may be a relationship between the time spent eating and sitting at the table and the amount of food needed to feel satisfied. Thin people tend to sit at the table for longer periods and pick at food, whereas the overweight eat large amounts at a faster rate.

items broiled or baked instead of fried? Are most of the dishes served with thick cheese or cream sauces? These are important things to know before you enter a restaurant—fast food or otherwise. Seafood restaurants usually offer broiled, baked, or poached fish, and you can often request butter and sauces on the side. Many steak houses offer small steaks and have salad bars.

NUTRITIONAL LABELS FOR RESTAURANTS

The nutrition facts panel on all supermarket foods became law in 1994. But because the content of menu items varies so much, and the menus in restaurants change so often, there is no labeling requirement for restaurants. However, since May 1997, if any restaurant makes a health claim about a food, such as that it is low-fat, the nutrition information has to comply with the meaning of that term, according to the Nutrition Labeling and Education Act (NLEA). Here are some of the facts behind restaurant claims:

Nutrition Claim	What It Means
Cholesterol-free	Less than 2 mg of cholesterol per serving
Fat-free	Less than 0.5 g of fat per serving
Sodium-free	Less than 5 mg of sodium per serving
Low-sodium	140 mg or less of sodium per seving
Sugar-free	Less than 0.5 g of sugar per serving
Low-sugar	May not be used as a claim

The term "healthy" when applied to a dish or other food item must describe a food low in saturated fat, with limited amounts of cholesterol and sodium, which provides significant amounts of key nutrients, such as vitamins A and C, iron, calcium, protein or fiber. If a restaurant makes a nutrition or health claim, it must provide you with that nutrition information when you request it. Don't be shy about asking: It's your health!

Try cuisines from other parts of the world. Italian and Asian restaurants often feature low-fat dishes—though you must be selective and alert so that large-sized portions do not sabotage your efforts. Try a small serving of pasta or fish in a meatless tomato sauce at an Italian restaurant. Many Chinese, Japanese, and Thai dishes include plenty of steamed vegetables, or a higher proportion of vegetables to meat than in American cuisine. Steamed rice, steamed noodle dishes, and vegetarian dishes are good choices too. When eating in an Asian restaurant, ask that the chef cook your food without soy sauce or salt to decrease the amount of sodium. (Many restaurant chefs will omit salt when requested.) Some Latin American restaurants feature a variety of fish and chicken dishes that are low in fat. If you enjoy Mexican cuisine, avoid cheese or sour cream sauces, or even dollops of sauce used as garnish, as they are often high in sodium. Don't be fooled by the rice in Mexican restaurants—it's usually cooked with oil and even lard.

Make sure you get what you want: Ask how dishes are cooked. Don't hesitate to request that one food be substituted for another. Order a green salad or baked potato in place of French fries. Order fruit, fruit ice, or sherbet instead of ice cream. Request sauces and salad dressing on the side and use only a minuscule amount. Better, squeeze some lemon or lime juice on

---

Fast Food Burgers

The burgers in most fast food restaurants are calorie- and fat-laden, but you can order the smallest size (not a Big Mac) and avoid the salty pickles for a special treat. Here are sample calorie counts:

McDonald's Hamburger: 260 calories   McDonald's Big Mac: 560 calories

Wendy's Jr. Hamburger: 270 calories   Wendy's Single: 360 calories

Hardee's Hamburger: 270 calories   Burger King Whopper: 640 calories

your greens. Ask that butter not be sent to the table with your breads or rolls. If you are not very hungry, order a low-fat appetizer rather than an entire meal, split a menu item with a friend, ask for a doggie bag and take half of your meat home, or order a half-size portion. When you have finished eating, ask the waiter to clear the dishes away that you can avoid post-meal nibbling.

Diets for Seniors

After the fifth decade of your life, you may notice that although you do not eat more than you used to, you keep putting on weight. This is because the rate at which your body converts food to energy slows about 2 percent every ten years. You don't need as much food as you did in your youth, but you do need as many nutrients. Another factor is the reduction of the amount of body mass (muscle is mostly protein) as you age. (Muscle mass burns more calories than fat does.) Since your body is making less protein, you need fewer calories than before. As you manage your diet, you should take some special care of your total health:

- Vitamin and mineral supplements can supply needed nutrients, especially if you eat small portions.

- Dairy products and orange juice are often supplemented with vitamin D. This vitamin is important for proper use of calcium by your body.

- Calcium is important to your bones; green leafy vegetables, milk, low-fat dairy products, and calcium-enriched breads can provide needed calcium. Your pharmacist can recommend a calcium supplement.

- When you eat less, you will have to drink more fluids because you are not getting the water that is in foods. So drink plenty of fluids, preferably water. If you are taking diuretics for HBP, this is especially important.

- Exercise daily. Be as active as possible in your daily life. You can slow the loss of muscle tone if you make sure you are as active as possible.

Calories No/Nutrition Yes

Most weight loss diets provide 1,200 to 2,000 calories per day. These are referred to as "low-calorie diets." However, the number of calories that is right for you depends on your weight, age, and activity level. If you have high blood pressure, your diet must be low-calorie to avoid adding weight and risking a rise in blood pressure. But it must also take into account your need to restrict salt intake, to boost your intake of fiber, and to limit the amount of fat, especially saturated fat (discussed in the next chapter), you consume. Your diet should allow for a weight loss of no more than one pound a week after the first week or two, when weight loss may be more rapid because of initial water loss. If you can estimate how many calories you eat in a day, you can design a diet and exercise strategy to lose about one-half to one pound a week. Or you can use a standardized low-calorie diet plan and adjust your calorie level.

Your diet should contain all the essential nutrients for your health. Use the Food Guide Pyramid (see page 112) and the Nutrition Facts label that is found on most processed food products (see pages 68–69 for a sample and explanation). The pyramid shows you the kinds and amounts of food that you need each day for good health. The Nutrition Facts label will help you select foods that meet your daily nutritional requirements. Make sure your diet includes:

Vitamins and Minerals: Eating a wide variety of foods from all food groups on the Food Guide Pyramid will ensure you get the vitamins and minerals you need. Select different foods, while staying within the basic guidelines. Eating a wide variety of foods also helps to provide a needed wide range of vitamins. If you eat less than 1,200 calories per day, you should take vitamin and mineral supplements.

Protein: The average woman who is over twenty-five years old should get 50 grams of protein daily, and the average man over twenty-five years of age should get 63 grams of protein daily. Protein prevents muscle tissue from breaking down and repairs body tissue such as skin and teeth. To get adequate protein in your diet, make sure you eat two to three servings from the meat, poultry, fish, dry beans, eggs, and nuts group on the Pyramid; all are good protein sources.

Carbohydrates: At least 100 grams of carbohydrates per day are needed to prevent fatigue and fluid imbalances. Eat six to eleven servings from the bread, cereal, rice, and pasta group shown in the pyramid. (Note: Each serving of carbohydrates is less than is normally served in a restaurant or home dish. You may be eating two servings of grains in just a snack. Remember, many carbohydrates are high in calories.)

Fiber: Adequate fiber helps with proper bowel function. If you were to eat 1 cup of bran cereal, one-half cup of carrots, one-half cup of kidney beans, a medium-sized pear, and a medium-sized apple in one day you should get about 30 grams of fiber.

Fat: Limit yourself to 30 percent of your calories, on average, from fat per day, with less than 10 percent of calories from saturated fat (fat from animal products such as meat, butter, and eggs). Limiting fat to these levels reduces the risk of heart disease and encourages weight loss. Also limit the amount of cholesterol, a fatlike substance (see next chapter) found in animal products such as meat, butter, and eggs. Your diet should include no more than 300 milligrams of cholesterol per day (for example, one egg contains about 215 milligrams of cholesterol and a hamburger contains about 100 milligrams of cholesterol).

Water: Eight glasses of water or water-based beverages every day. You may need more water if you exercise a lot.

These nutrients should come from a variety of low-calorie, nutrient-rich foods. One way to get variety is to choose foods each day from the Food Pyramid.

Exercise Makes a Diet Work

Everybody has always told you that exercise helps you lose those extra pounds. And everybody was right. Regular activity helps you lose weight, and does a great deal more. It helps you feel and look better and it also helps to lower high blood pressure. Almost any kind of activity can accomplish a weight loss; you don't have to run a marathon to benefit from exercise. Any activity, if done at least thirty minutes a day over the course of a long time, will make a difference. (For more about exercise, see Chapter 29.)

Since your weight depends on a balance between the calories you take in and those you use up, you need to use both ends against your middle (pun intended). Increase your exercise as you decrease your calories. Begin by determining how many calories you are taking in daily. Next, study the table on page 113 to get an idea of the number of calories used up in various forms of exercise.

You will very quickly be able to see the relationship between what you are taking in and how much you are working off. It won't be hard to under-

FOOD GUIDE PYRAMID
A Guide to Daily Food Choices

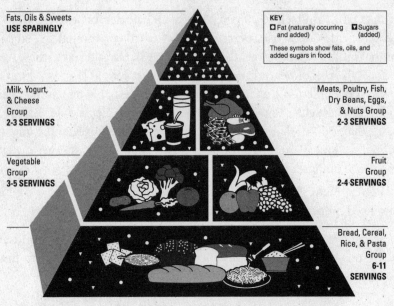

Fats, Oils & Sweets
USE SPARINGLY

KEY
☐ Fat (naturally occurring   ▼ Sugars
   and added)   (added)

These symbols show fats, oils, and
added sugars in food.

Milk, Yogurt,
& Cheese
Group
2-3 SERVINGS

Meats, Poultry, Fish,
Dry Beans, Eggs,
& Nuts Group
2-3 SERVINGS

Vegetable
Group
3-5 SERVINGS

Fruit
Group
2-4 SERVINGS

Bread, Cereal,
Rice, & Pasta
Group
**6-11
SERVINGS**

Source: U.S. Department of Agriculture &
U.S. Department of Health and Human Services

stand why if you are sedentary and have a big appetite, you just keep putting on weight. Once you really understand how much exercise you need to do to burn up just a few calories, you may come to the conclusion that one of the best exercises is pushing away from the table.

Other Weight Loss Tactics

There are other, extreme methods of losing weight. I don't recommend any of them, but here they are for the sake of completion. Healthy diet and moderate exercise are always to be preferred.

Behavior modification is based on the experiments of Pavlov, a Russian psychologist whose experiments conditioned a dog to salivate on hearing a bell because the dog had been trained to know that a bell sounded when he was to be fed. In dietary behavior modification, food is associated

---

Exercise Burns Calories

Here is how much you have to exercise to make up for indulging in fattening foods:

Burning off one 3½ ounce glass of dry white wine (85 calories) requires:

 6 minutes of running 7.5 miles per hour for a loss of 13.2 calories per minute

 22 minutes of walking 3 miles per hour for a loss of 3.8 calories per minute

 10 minutes of swimming for a loss of 8.1 calories per minute

Burning off one fried egg (115 calories) requires:

 9 minutes of running

 30 minutes of walking

 14 minutes of swimming

Burning off one cola (145 calories) requires:

 11 minutes of running

 38 minutes of walking

 18 minutes of swimming

---

with a small electric shock or some other type of unpleasant response. People who have stayed with this type of therapy have found it successful. However, it is time-consuming and unpleasant.

The reward approach can also be applied to dieting. I have two friends, physicians and partners, who have agreed to pay each other a dollar reward for each pound of weight loss either can show. Unfortunately, so far this has not worked too well, and neither has lost much weight. I believe the problem here is that motivation is basic to weight loss, and this type of external encouragement is insufficient.

Psychotherapy, both in groups and individually, has been tried with limited success, as has hypnosis, but results have not been impressive.

Surgery has been used for morbidly obese people; it can block off part of the stomach or shorten the intestinal tract so that the passageway ab-

Activity Ideas

Take a walk

Get off the bus one or two stops early

Ride a bike

Clean your house

Go bowling or play tennis

Play with children or a pet

Use the stairs

Park far away from your destination

Work in the yard or garden

Put on the radio and dance

Carry your own groceries

Use a push mower to cut the grass

sorbs less food. This drastic method of controlling food intake has had some excellent results.

Whether you are overweight or not, regular exercise (at least three times a week) is important to look and feel your best, and keep you blood pressure within the normal range. If you do need to lose weight, stepping up your activity level will cause you to burn calories more quickly and help make weight loss easier.

Don't Forget Your Nutritional Needs

It's easy to lose sight of your body's nutritional requirements while you focus on weight loss. When choosing "thin" foods that help you diet, don't forget about your energy requirements, your body type, age, and overall health as well as special conditions, such as pregnancy. Your caloric needs and therefore the effects of a decreased caloric intake must be discussed with your doctor.

Since everyone is different, the weight loss methods that work for one will not necessarily work for another. However, here are the basic guidelines that will enable you to keep your weight down and remain healthy:

The Ten Nutrition Commandments

Following are ten commandments that, if followed, will lead to good nutritional health:

Thou shalt not eat an unbalanced or unvaried diet.

Thou shalt not disregard the calorie count—keep it sacred.

Thou shalt change eating habits.

Thou shalt listen to internal body signals and eat only when hunger is felt.

Thou shalt not eat because of social, emotional, or enticement pressures.

Thou shall not eat incorrect foods, only correct ones.

Thou shalt not eat too much salt or sugar.

Thou shalt not eat too much cholesterol or saturated fat.

Thou shalt not drink too much alcohol.

Thou shalt increase the number of fiber foods.

CHAPTER 12

Cholesterol As a Culprit

Not only is high blood pressure a leading cause of heart disease, but an important connection has been found between hypertension and an elevated cholesterol level. To avoid or manage hypertension, you must avoid as much cholesterol in foods as possible or manage your cholesterol levels if they become elevated.

Cholesterol Clogs Your Arteries

When there is too much cholesterol in your blood, the excess can become trapped in the walls of your arteries. Building up along the walls of the arteries that supply blood to the heart, cholesterol is a major factor causing so-called hardening of the arteries, or atherosclerosis. The cholesterol buildup narrows the arteries, slowing or even blocking the flow of blood to the heart muscle.

Ever since medical experts have found that dietary fats are related to heart disease, classifying fats has become complicated. There are different kinds of fats, some of which are worse for our arteries than others. And recently, researchers have found that some fats may actually be good for your arteries. In addition to saturated fat (which is solid at room temperature, like the fat on a thick steak) and unsaturated fat (the golden liquid in a bottle of olive oil), there are triglycerides, trans fatty acids, and omega-3 and omega-6 fatty acids. Almost every day, we hear new reports and changing recommendations about what to eat and what not to eat. One day, we hear

> ### Debra's Arteries Can't Stand the Pressure
>
> Debra was sprinting for a bus when she suddenly felt a sharp pain, as if someone were squeezing their arms hard around her chest. As she staggered under this crushing sensation, she began having trouble breathing. She could not draw in enough air. When Debra collapsed, a passerby noticed and called the police. Moments later, a medical team arrived. As soon as Debra was in the EMS ambulance, paramedics used an electrocardiograph, which revealed that one area of her heart no longer produced a normal electrical pattern. This area, cut off from its blood supply, was dead. Debra had coronary heart disease (CHD). A thickening inside the walls of the coronary arteries (atherosclerosis) had produced Debra's heart attack.

that lard is bad, and that margarine is better than butter. The next day, we hear the exact opposite.

FAT-RELATED VOCABULARY

Cholesterol: A soft, waxy substance. The body makes enough cholesterol to meet its needs. Cholesterol is used in the manufacture of hormones, bile acid, and vitamin D. It is present in all parts of the body, including the nervous system, muscle, skin, liver, intestines, and heart.

—*Blood cholesterol:* Cholesterol circulating in the bloodstream. It is made in the liver and also absorbed from the food you eat. The blood carries it to all parts of the body. A high level of blood cholesterol leads to atherosclerosis and an increased risk of heart disease.

—*Dietary cholesterol:* The cholesterol in the food you eat. It is present only in foods of animal origin, not those of plant origin. Dietary cholesterol, like dietary saturated fat, raises blood cholesterol, which increases the risk for heart disease.

Fat: A chemical compound containing one or more fatty acids. Fat is the principal form in which energy is stored in the body.

Fatty acid: The building blocks of fat.

Hydrogenated fat: Fat in liquid form that is chemically altered to become solid. Vegetable shortening and margarine are examples.

Lipid: A chemical compound that is insoluble in water. Both fat and cholesterol are lipids.

Lipoprotein: A compound made of fat and protein. Lipids have more fat than protein. Lipoproteins have more protein than fat. Lipoproteins are found in blood cholesterol.

High-density lipoprotein (HDL): This is the so-called good cholesterol.

Low-density lipoprotein (LDL): The so-called bad cholesterol. LDLs carry most of the cholesterol in the blood. The cholesterol and fat from LDLs are the main source of dangerous buildup and blockage in the arteries. The more LDL cholesterol you have in your blood, the greater the risk of cholesterol buildup in your arteries.

Monounsaturated fatty acids: Fatty acids that are found mostly in plants and seafoods. Olive oil and canola (rapeseed) oil are high in monounsaturated fatty acids, which tend to lower levels of LDL in the blood.

Polyunsaturated fatty acids: Fatty acids that are low in hydrogen atoms. Safflower oil and corn oil are high in polyunsaturated fatty acids, which tend to lower levels of both HDL and LDL cholesterol in the blood.

Saturated fatty acids: Found in meat, whole milk, butter, and lard, saturated fatty acids tend to raise levels of LDL cholesterol in the blood.

Trans fatty acids: A polyunsaturated fatty acid that becomes solid through a process called hydrogenation.

Triglycerides: Lipids carried through the bloodstream to tissues. Most of the body's fat tissue is in the form of triglycerides, stored for use as energy. Triglycerides come from fat in foods.

Cholesterol is a soapy, yellowish white type of fat that is essential for body-building. It is found in bile (produced by the liver), in the insulation of the nerves, and as a component of androgen (the male sex hormone) and estrogen (the female sex hormone). Cholesterol is a sort of cousin of fat. Both fat and cholesterol belong to a larger family of chemical compounds called lipids. All the cholesterol your body needs is made by your liver.

Cholesterol is used to build cell membranes and your body's tissues. People don't need to consume dietary cholesterol, because the body makes enough for its needs.

The typical American diet contains substantial amounts of unneeded cholesterol. It is found in egg yolks, liver, meat, some shellfish, and whole milk dairy products. Saturated fat associated with high cholesterol is usually not found in vegetable products, but coconut oil, palm oil, and cocoa butter have high amounts of saturated fatty acids. About 25 percent of the cholesterol in the body comes from what we eat.

Serum cholesterol, blood cholesterol, and total cholesterol all mean almost the same thing—the cholesterol in your body. This is what is measured when you have a cholesterol test.

Lowering Dietary Fat Lowers Cholesterol

I recommend that fats make up only 30 percent of your total caloric intake. Some heart and hypertension experts suggest even lower levels. Either way, these levels are substantially lower than the levels in most American diets. Cutting fat intake levels has a dramatic effect on reducing high blood pressure.

A diet high in saturated fat increases blood cholesterol because your liver transforms it into cholesterol. To decrease your blood cholesterol level, you must decrease saturated fat in your diet. (Unsaturated fat does not convert to cholesterol, but actually reduces blood cholesterol levels.) Some dietary fat is needed for good health. Fats supply energy and essential fatty acids and promote absorption of the fat-soluble vitamins A, D, E, and K. Because of public awareness programs sponsored by the American Heart Association and other organizations such as the National Institutes of Health, most Americans know that they should eat less saturated fat and cholesterol-rich foods. However, many people continue to eat high-fat diets, and obesity is epidemic. Paradoxically, despite all the news concerning the dangers of high-saturated-fat diets, the average weight has gone up. Some nutritionists believe that counting fat grams is as important as counting calories.

Review the Food Guide Pyramid (page 112). Some foods in each group have a higher fat content than others. Choose foods lower in fat among the foods in each group. This allows you to eat the recommended servings from these groups. You also get to increase the amount and variety of grain

Maximum Fat Intake for Calorie Levels

Calorie intake	1,600	2,200	2,800
Total fat (grams)	53	73	93

products, fruits, and vegetables in your diet without adding to your calorie count.

HDL to the Rescue

HDL is shorthand for the high-density lipoproteins that help your body in its battle with cholesterol. Low-density lipoproteins (LDLs) are composed mainly of cholesterol. Therefore, they can lead to a fatty buildup in the arteries. High-density lipoproteins (HDLs) are mainly protein, however; their action resists the formation of cholesterol in the body and draws the cholesterol away from the walls of the arteries. Although differences of opinion about the role and importance of HDL exist among medical and nutritional experts, there seems to be agreement on the following points:

- HDL is low in some people, which may lead to cholesterol-clogged arteries.
- HDL is high in some people, which may account for low cholesterol levels in those people.
- Exercise will increase the level of HDL.

When your cholesterol is checked, laboratories give you a number called a cholesterol ratio. This number is your total cholesterol rating divided by your HDL level. Combining the two levels into one number gives you a view of your risk for several diseases. But the ratio is general. It is important to know the value for each level, because LDL and HDL cholesterol both determine your health risks.

How Does LDL Obstruct Blood Circulation?

When LDL cholesterol is oxidized by free radicals it forms plaque, which causes artery blockage. A free radical is a molecular fragment that has an unpaired electron. Whenever LDL particles are exposed to these unstable molecules, the LDL particles are oxidized (like oxidized iron particles—rust—which are bumpy and rough). They also become stickier, which increases the risk of the formation of a blood clot. An oxidized LDL particle becomes toxic to the human body.

Nonoxidized LDL is recognized as "self" or nonthreatening by the body's immune system. But oxidized LDL is so changed that our immune system identifies it as "nonself" and potentially dangerous. To guard the body from this perceived outsider, the immune system's large scavenger cells engulf and swallow the oxidized LDLs. These LDL-bloated scavenger cells then gather in tiny cracks or injuries in the artery walls, where they embed themselves and protrude into the artery, clogging it.

What Are Triglycerides?

Triglycerides are the form in which fat is carried through your blood and to the tissues. The bulk of your body's fat tissue is in the form of triglycerides. Your triglycerides are measured whenever your LDL cholesterol is checked. Triglyceride levels less than 200 mg/dl (milligrams per deciliter) are considered normal.

It is not clear whether high triglycerides alone increase your risk of heart disease. But many people with high triglycerides also have high LDL or low HDL levels, which do increase the risk of heart disease.

Low-Cholesterol Cultures

After World War II, medical researchers in Scandinavia noticed that deaths from heart disease had declined when food was rationed and when meat,

Selecting Low-Cholesterol Foods

The most important rule for any healthy eating plan is to keep your daily intake of cholesterol under 300 milligrams and to keep the percent of calories you get from fat under 30. This doesn't mean you have to starve. See the chart in Appendix 3, pages 325–31, which lists many popular foods. The chart also includes the number of calories and the sodium content in those foods. You may want to duplicate this chart and carry it with you.

dairy products, and eggs were scarce. Since then, it has been found that in countries where the average person's cholesterol level is less than 180 mg/dl, very few people develop atherosclerosis. In the United States, where average levels are above 220 mg/dl, heart disease is the leading cause of death. But high-fat diets and high rates of disease don't always go together.

People living on the Greek island of Crete have very low rates of heart disease, even though olive oil is a big part of their diet. They consume high levels of HDL cholesterol. The Inuit people of Alaska and Greenland also are mostly free of clogged artery disease despite a high-fat, high-cholesterol diet. A diet staple for the Inuit is fish rich in omega-3 polyunsaturated fatty acids. Vegetable sources for omega-3 oils are flax seeds and primrose, soybean, and olive oils. Fish sources such as salmon and mackerel lower LDL cholesterol and triglyceride levels in the blood.

Omega-6 polyunsaturated fatty acids have also been found in some studies to reduce both LDL and HDL cholesterol levels in the blood. Linoleic acid, an essential nutrient and a component of corn, soybean, and safflower oils, is an omega-6 fatty acid.

Choose a Diet Low in Fat

Fat, whether from plant or animal sources, contains more than twice the number of calories of an equal amount of carbohydrate or protein. Choose a diet that provides no more than 30 percent of total calories from fat. The upper limit on the grams of fat in your diet will depend on the calories you need. Cutting back on fat may help you consume fewer calories. For example, at 2,000 calories a day, the suggested upper limit of calories from fat is about 600 calories (65 grams of fat $\times$ 9 calories per gram = about 600 calories).

Margarine vs. Butter

You may have heard that margarine has a type of unsaturated fat called trans fatty acids. These fats appear to raise blood cholesterol more than other unsaturated fats, but not as much as saturated fats. Trans fatty acids are formed when vegetable oil is hardened or hydrogenated to make margarine or shortening. The harder the margarine or shortening, the more likely it is to contain these trans fatty acids. Read the ingredients label. Choose margarine containing liquid vegetable oil as the first ingredient rather than hydrogenated or partially hydrogenated oil. Use the nutrition labels to choose margarine with the least amount of saturated fat. Tip: A friend has devised a way of cutting fat in spreads even more. She buys a softened partially saturated spread. She then beats in about a half cup of skim milk. She recools the spread; it goes on smoothly, with fewer calories and less saturated fat.

Fat Labels

Here are the main label claims used on food packages and what they mean.

SATURATED FAT

- Saturated fat free: Less than one-half gram of saturated fat in a serving. Trans fatty acids must be not more than 12 percent of total fat.
- Low saturated fat: 1 gram or less of saturated fat in a serving and 15 percent or less of the total calories from saturated fat. A meal or main dish (for example, a frozen dinner) should include 1 gram of saturated fat or less per 100 grams of food, and less than 10 percent of the total calories from saturated fat.

CHOLESTEROL

- Cholesterol free: Less than 2 milligrams of cholesterol in a serving; the saturated fat content must be 2 grams or less.
- Low cholesterol: 20 milligrams or less of cholesterol in a serving. Saturated fat content must be 2 grams or less. A meal or main dish should include 20 milligrams or less of cholesterol per 100 grams of food, and less than 2 grams of saturated fat in 100 grams of food.

FAT

- Fat free: Less than one-half gram of fat in a serving.
- Low fat: 3 grams total fat or less in a serving. A meal or main dish should include 3 grams or less of total fat in 100 grams of food and less than 30 percent calories from fat.
- Percent fat free: A food with this claim must also meet the low-fat claim.

CALORIES

- Calorie free: Less than 5 calories in a serving.
- Low calorie: 40 calories or less in a serving.

Lite/Light and Lean

We've all seen products that announce how "light" or "lite" they are. We assume that means that the product has a low fat content. Are these just meaningless words used in advertising? What do they really mean?

- Light: A product with half the fat or one-third fewer calories than the regular product.

- Reduced/less/lower/fewer: A food (like a lower fat hot dog) with at least 25 percent less calories, fat, saturated fat, cholesterol, or sodium than the regular product.

- Lean: Less than 10 grams of fat, 4.5 grams of saturated fat, and 95 milligrams of cholesterol in a serving of meat, poultry, fish, or shellfish.

- Extra lean: Less than 5 grams of fat, 2 grams of saturated fat, and 95 milligrams of cholesterol in a serving of meat, poultry, or shellfish. Warning: Some products that advertise "reduced-fat" or "reduced calories" are actually smaller versions of the product. A "reduced-fat" candy bar might just be smaller than the regular bar.

Phony Fats

Low-fat cookies, nonfat spreads, even fat-free cheese—how do they do it? And what are you eating? The genius of food technology has devised fat-free-based replacements for high-fat foods. Carbohydrate- and protein-based fakes, such as carrageenan, guar gum, and whey protein mimic the feel of fat in your mouth. Here are some of the new substitutes (always check labels).

- Appetize: 9 calories per gram. It is made of animal fats with the cholesterol removed; in shortening and in margarine, it is used in commercial products.

- Fruit or vegetable puree: Usually less than 3 calories per gram: Prune butter, apple sauce, or other purees can be used in baked goods. A plus is that these provide fiber in the diet.

- Hydrolyzed oat flour: About 1 calorie per gram. Made from oat flour treated with an enzyme, it has a creamy texture. Used in dressings, soups, and sauces. It lowers cholesterol and provides some fiber.

- Olestra (Olean): 0 calories per gram. Made from combining vegetable oil and sugar, it cannot be absorbed by the body. The Food and Drug Administration has approved it, but there are many side effects, among them diarrhea. Olestra reduces the absorption of foods eaten with it.

- Salatrim: 5 calories per gram. This product is made with various fatty acids. It cannot be used in fried foods, and is often used in chocolate-flavored foods.

- Simplese: 4 calories per gram. A protein product that is used in sauces, baked foods, and frozen desserts.

- Xenical: Approved by the FDA in 1999, this is a pill that has no calories and blocks about 30 percent of the fat that you eat in other foods. Side effects include a change in bowel habits.

Note: There isn't anything wrong with fruit or vegetable purees, but I reserve judgment on the other products. Each has some side effect which may not be pleasant.

Guilt-Free Restaurant Fare

You can enjoy a wonderful meal in almost any restaurant. But you may have to speak up and ask your waiter questions. Ask for lean cuts of red meats, fish, or chicken. Then ask how the entrée is prepared: avoid fried, breaded, or sauced meat dishes. Request broiled, grilled, or poached meats, fish, or poultry. Here are some other tips:

- Become a fat-finder: When you eat out, seek out fat. Watch out for butter, cream, sour cream, cheese, avocado, and sausages. Mexican chimichangas, broccoli smothered with cheese sauce, or stuffed potato skins are no-nos.

- Breads can be avoided, or eaten without butter. Try dark or grainy breads (pumpernickel, rye, or wheat) and hard rolls high in fiber. Avoid croissants, biscuits, and muffins.

- Cheese or cheese sauces are often high in saturated fat. Cheese-based salad dressings and mayonnaise are often higher in fat than a broiled chicken breast. Add pepper and herbs to make the food really tasty. Ask that all salad dressings and sauces be on the side. Use them sparingly.

- Choose clear soups rather than cream soups, and avoid any cheese-based soup. (Unfortunately, many soups are very high in salt.)

- Pasta is great, but look for tomato-based sauces without meat. Avoid creamy sauces such as Alfredo or parmigiana. Learn to modify dishes that seem too heavily sauced by scraping off the extra sauce. (Tip: Place fatty meats on a piece of bread. The fat will drain into the bread as you cut the meat. Never eat the bread.)

- Order an appetizer and eat it as your meal. Most restaurant meals will provide a day's worth of cholesterol, fats, and salt. Take a doggie bag home if you order a full meal. Become friends with your wait-person, and he or she will understand. You're not the first person to avoid too much fat.

Teens love to eat with their friends, and most teens love fast food. You'll find a section on fast foods in the fats table on page 331, in Appendix 3. But that information is just a start. Restaurants change their menus and introduce new foods every few months. Familiarize yourself with the menu of your teen's local hangout and check with the restaurant for the nutritional analysis of the foods served. Teens are very body-aware and they will be interested in the fat and calorie count of various offerings. A grilled chicken sandwich is a better choice than a hamburger. And a plain burger is obviously better than a bacon burger or a cheeseburger. If your teen seems interested, suggest salads with no dressing or just a drizzle of low-fat dressing. Most of all, be a good example yourself.

CHAPTER 13

Fiber Is Important

Our grandparents called it "bulk" or "roughage," but now the popular name is "fiber." It is the stuff that puts the crunch in carrots, the bulk in salads, the chew in whole grain bread, and the thickening in the stewed prunes and pea soup. Unfortunately, Americans don't eat enough of it.

What Is Fiber?

Fiber in the diet is a diverse group of chemical compounds including cellulose, hemicelluloses, pectins, gums, and lignin. All of these, except lignin, are complex carbohydrates, very tough substances found in plants. Some fibers, like cellulose, are components of wood, as well as edible plants. These are rough, fibrous, and insoluble in water. Pectins and gums are water-soluble and form gel-like textures. Pectin, for instance, makes jelly gel. The amount of edible fiber varies from plant to plant. The stalk of the broccoli plant contains more fiber than the flowers, and generally the older a plant is, the more fiber it contains.

What can fiber do for you? Studies link diets low in saturated fats and cholesterol, but high in fiber, with reduced risks of several serious diseases, including cardiovascular disease. Adequate fiber intake also decreases the transit time of food traveling through the digestive tract. Faster transit time means less contact with the natural toxins within body waste and a reduced risk of colon problems. Fiber absorbs water, adds bulk, and softens stool; with less straining required to pass a softer stool, the probability of developing hemorrhoids is reduced.

Take It Slow

A word of caution: When increasing the fiber content of your diet, it's best to take it slow. Add just a few grams at a time to allow the intestinal tract to adjust. Otherwise you may experience cramps, gas, bloating, diarrhea, or constipation. Other ways to help minimize such effects:

◆ Drink about 8 cups of water daily.

◆ Don't cook dried beans in the same water you used for soaking the beans.

◆ Use enzyme products such as Beano or Say Yes to Beans to help digest fiber.

Fiber binds cholesterol and liver bile in the digestive tract, preventing its recirculation in the bloodstream. Fiber can the lower blood cholesterol levels. Fiber also binds and reduces the absorption of dietary fat, which can be helpful in weight control.

Fiber is also key in weight loss: Because insoluble fiber is indigestible and passes through the body virtually intact, it provides few calories. And since the digestive tract can handle only a small amount of bulk at a time, fiber-rich foods are more filling than other foods—so people tend to eat less.

The Food and Drug Administration has recognized the importance of fiber by requiring it to be listed on the Nutrition Facts panel of food labels along with other key nutrients and calories. Dietary soluble fiber, when part of a diet low in saturated fat and low cholesterol, may reduce the risk of coronary heart disease.

High Blood Pressure and Fiber

Most important for anyone with HBP, fiber may be a key to keeping pressure down without medication. James A. Anderson, a physician working at the Veterans Administration Medical Center in Lexington, Kentucky, placed twelve men on a fourteen-day diet that contained three times as much dietary fiber as a control diet, and the average blood pressure in this control group dropped 10 percent. In other patients whose blood pressure had been normal, systolic pressure was lowered 8 percent and diastolic pressure dropped about 10 percent.

FIBER FOODS

It is sensible to include healthy amounts of fiber in the foods we eat. But just how much is a "healthy amount"? Dietary experts recommend that we aim for about 20 to 25 grams of fiber each day, also advising that we eat several servings of foods that contain fiber each day. Try to get at least one or two servings of the following into your daily diet.

Fruits:

| blackberries | raspberries | strawberries | figs | |
| raisins | prunes | dates | pears | apples |

Cereals and grains:

| bran breads | oat breads | pumpernickel bread |
| bran cereals | oat cereals | oat bran cereals |

Dried beans and peas:

| broad beans | black beans | pinto beans | |
| navy beans | chickpeas | lentils | split peas |

Tip: When it is practical, eat well-washed fruits and vegetables with their skins.

There are several types of fiber: Fruits are a source of pectins, particularly citrus fruits and apples. Cellulose is common in all plants, but there is more in the outer layers of cereal grains and the tough fibrous parts of fruits, vegetables, and legumes. Starchy foods such as cereals have fiber too. In addition to fiber, foods from roots such as carrots and potatoes contain needed nutrients.

The Downside

Don't go overboard in consuming fiber. Besides causing bloating and gas, excess fiber can prevent your body from absorbing such minerals as calcium, zinc, copper, and selenium. Too much dietary fiber may lead to deficiencies in these trace minerals. Any attempt to increase fiber consumption above usual levels should be undertaken gradually. Individual tolerance and need for fiber varies.

CHAPTER 14

Sugar Is Not Sweet to Your Body

With all the low-fat food products on the market, it seems ironic that Americans are actually getting fatter and fatter all the time. Obesity rates in children are also increasing. My guess is that people, in their efforts to cut down on fats, are turning to sugar. That high-fiber bran muffin without butter tastes better with more jelly.

Sugars are carbohydrates. Dietary carbohydrates also include the complex carbohydrates starch and fiber. During digestion, all carbohydrates except fiber break down into sugars. Sugars and starches occur naturally in many foods such as milk, fruits, some vegetables, breads, cereals, and grains. Americans eat sugars in many forms, and as small children we grow to like their taste. Some sugars are used as natural preservatives, thickeners, and baking aids in foods; they are often added to foods during processing and preparation, or when they are eaten. The body cannot tell the difference between naturally occurring and added refined sugars, because they are identical chemically.

Sugar and Weight Maintenance

Contrary to popular belief, scientific evidence indicates that diets high in sugars do not cause hyperactivity or diabetes. The most common type of diabetes occurs in overweight people. Avoiding sugars alone will not correct being overweight. To lose weight, reduce the total amount of calories from the food you eat and increase your level of physical activity.

If you wish to maintain your weight when you eat less fat, replace the

---

Sweet Facts

According to the Department of Nutrition and Food Studies at New York University, consumption of sugars and other caloric sweeteners has risen 28 percent between 1983 and 1999. In the United States more than half of these sweeteners come from soft drinks, baked goods, and fruit drinks. In 1977, the average American ate 1,854 calories a day; by 1996, the daily calorie intake rose to 2,002. The percentage of obese adults rose from 25 to 35 percent.

---

lost calories from fat with equal calories from fruits, vegetables, and grain products, which you can find in the lower half of the Food Guide Pyramid. Some foods that contain a lot of sugars supply calories but few or no nutrients. These foods are located at the top of the pyramid. For athletes and active people with high calorie needs, sugars can be an additional source of energy.

Because maintaining a nutritious diet and a healthy weight is very important in controlling HBP, sugars should be used sparingly by people with low calorie needs. Avoid eating lots of sugars and sugary snacks. Most sugar substitutes do not provide significant calories and therefore may be useful in low-calorie diets. Foods containing sugar substitutes such as sorbitol, saccharin, and aspartame, however, may not always be lower in calories than similar products that contain sugars. Some people have strong adverse reactions to aspartame. Unless you reduce the total calories you eat, then the use of sugar substitutes cannot be a magic formula for weight loss.

Sweet Drinks Count

Sodas are the largest single source of added sugars, according to a recent study. In one 12-ounce can of soda there are 10 teaspoons of added sugar. A higher percentage of 12- to 29-year-old people drink soda regularly than any other group. Men and boys average about two cans a day, women and girls average about one and a half cans. People apparently ignore all the excess calories they consume as liquids. Instead of sugar, try lemon, which is a great flavor-maker; carbonated water, without added salt, or plain water with a slice of lemon may satisfy your thirst and your desire for a taste sensation.

Sugar on a Food Label

Learn to identify sugar under its various guises:

brown sugar	corn sweetener	corn syrup	fructose
juice concentrate	glucose	dextrose	maltose
fructose corn syrup	honey	invert sugar	lactose
molasses	raw sugar	syrup	sucrose

Researchers at Georgetown University Medical Center in Washington, D.C., tested the effects of a high-sugar diet on blood pressure in hypertensive rats. They found that such a diet markedly increased the rats' blood pressure in only two weeks. Most important, the high blood pressure was reversible with a low-sugar diet. When Richard A. Ahrens, at the University of Maryland, duplicated this study with human subjects, the results were the same. Sugar can also contribute to sodium retention and thus contribute to higher blood pressure.

CHAPTER 15

Diabetes and Kidney Disease and Hypertension

About 14 million Americans are affected with diabetes and will need treatment for life. As with hypertensives, self-management is recommended as a way of taking control of diabetes. Through self-management, diabetics can often keep their blood sugar levels within a healthy range.

Diabetes—Its Causes and Symptoms

Insulin is a natural hormone produced by the pancreas. It enables the cells in the body to take in sugars and either use them immediately for quick energy, or store them in the body for an even level of energy output. Diabetes occurs when the body is insulin-deficient or becomes impaired in its capacity to use insulin, or both.

Some of the common symptoms of diabetes include: extreme thirst, frequent urination, hunger, dry skin, slow healing, fatigue, headaches, vision problems, sweating, rapid heartbeat, and even trembling. Proper blood sugar and insulin control can prevent or lessen these problems.

Diabetes and Hypertension

High blood pressure is common in people with diabetes. Native Americans, Hispanics, and African-Americans all have increased risk of having both diseases. Moreover, once you develop diabetes, your odds for devel-

---

Omega-3 Fatty Acids Do Good Once Again

In a recent Italian study, diets high in omega-3 fatty acids have shown benefits to subjects with diabetes. The fatty oils seem to change lipid metabolism
while lowering high blood pressure and reducing cardiovascular risk factors.
No downside here!

---

oping high blood pressure increase. Between 35 and 75 percent of all complications associated with diabetes can be attributed to hypertension.

Hypertension and diabetes are interrelated diseases. If either of these
diseases is untreated, the patient will be vulnerable to both atherosclerotic
cardiovascular disease and renal disease. More than three million Americans have both hypertension and diabetes. Both diseases respond well to
weight management programs that prescribe salt reduction, moderate alcohol intake, increased physical activity, and quitting smoking.

Exercise Reduces Diabetes

In the fall of 1999, the results of the Nurses Health Study of more than seventy thousand women were reported. Researchers found that exercise can
reduce the risk of developing diabetes, as well as improve heart and vascular health. The most vigorous exercise was associated with a 46 percent
lower risk for diabetes; even brisk walking showed significant benefits.

Over-the-Counter Medication Interactions
if You Have Diabetes and HBP

Avoid decongestants that are taken by mouth. These products can raise
your blood glucose and should be used only if recommended by your doctor. As always, study all labels; they can be useful. If you see the caution
statement, "Individuals with high blood pressure, heart disease, or diabetes
should use only as directed by physician," on the label of a nonprescription
drug you are considering, don't buy it until you consult your doctor: It is
important to take this alert seriously.

High Blood Pressure and Kidney Disease

Throughout the day, the blood in your body flows through your kidneys, which filter the blood and excrete waste products through your urine. The kidneys are vital to your health by preventing toxic waste products and extra fluid from building up. Your blood pressure is related to the health of your kidneys; high blood pressure can damage the kidneys.

As we've discussed, high blood pressure makes the heart work harder, and over time can damage blood vessels throughout the body. If the blood vessels in the kidneys are damaged, the kidneys may stop doing their job. Extra fluid then may accumulate, raising blood pressure even more. After diabetes, high blood pressure is the leading cause of kidney failure, commonly called end-stage renal disease (ESRD). Patients with ESRD must either go on dialysis or receive a new kidney through a transplant. Every year, high blood pressure causes more than fifteen thousand new cases of ESRD in the United States.

Creatinine, a by-product of muscle breakdown, is a colorless nonmineral crystal found in the blood. Elevated blood levels of creatinine are generally linked to impaired kidney function. This raises a special warning flag for people with high blood pressure, as it signals a risk for heart attack or stroke. Hypertensive people should ask their doctors about their creatinine level. For more information contact: the American Kidney Fund, 6110 Executive Boulevard, Rockville, MD 20852 (800-638-8299) or the National Kidney Foundation, 30 East 33rd Street, New York, NY 10016 (800-622-9010).

Renal Hypertension

For many years, physicians have known that clamping the renal artery in animals resulted in hypertension. It is now known that any interference with the blood supply to the human kidney causes excess production of renin, which as we have seen causes hypertension. If the blood supply to the kidney can be restored, renin is no longer produced and the hypertension is relieved.

Such a case of blood pressure is called renal hypertension. Unfortunately, it is almost impossible to tell renal hypertension from the usual type. The blood pressure readings are no different, and there is no simple screening test. There is only one physical sign that uniquely points to renal

> ### Dangerous Driving
>
> When I was a physician in the emergency room of St. Vincent's Hospital in New York City, I was called to examine a truck driver who had left his eighteen-wheeler right outside the emergency room door. The teamster complained that he "just didn't feel right." Blood tests revealed severe uremia. It is surprising that he was able to do it, but he had driven across the country. Uremia is a silent and extremely dangerous condition.

hypertension—a roaring sound caused by blood flowing through a constricted artery. That sound can be heard with a stethoscope.

Renal hypertension is most frequent in men over the age of 50. Researchers are developing various surgical techniques to open up or bypass clogged renal arteries. The present theory is that a person may be better off without a damaged kidney that is causing high blood pressure.

Hypertensive Retinopathy

The retina is the innermost lining of the eye. It receives images formed by the lens and is the instrument of vision. High blood pressure can cause the retinal blood vessels to constrict, resulting in vision loss. The longer the duration of hypertension, the more damage to the eye's blood vessels. This is yet one more risk of untreated or poorly controlled hypertension.

If you suffer HBP and notice headaches with visual disturbances, alert your doctor. Through the ophthalmoscope, he or she will look into your eyes, looking for small retinal hemorrhages. Early detection and control of hypertension may be the best way of looking at . . . everything.

Answers to Questions About Weight, Hypertension, and Diabetes

The combination of diet, exercise, self-monitoring and drugs, when prescribed by your doctor, has greatly increased the survival and well-being of people with diabetes, people with high blood pressure, and people with both. Here are the two questions my patients who have both diseases have often asked:

Can a person who is very overweight with diabetes and hypertension completely eliminate symptoms of both diseases by losing weight through diet and exercise?

It is possible for some people, especially those who have mild cases of either or both diseases and who are consistent in their efforts, to lose weight. In some studies of diabetes, it appears that if an obese person who recently developed diabetes begins to lose pounds, his sensitivity to insulin increases even before he attains his ideal weight. Alas, if the disease has persisted for many years, shedding pounds may not be sufficient to overcome either or both diseases.

Do people of normal weight who have a low-fat, low-calorie diet still have a higher risk of developing diabetes if one of their parents had diabetes or high blood pressure?

It has long been recognized that hypertension seems to "run in some families." Recently, science has discovered that genetic factors may also play a role in diabetes. Those with a strong family history of either disease need to be extra vigilant about their diet and cardiovascular fitness. They may be able to reduce their elevated risk of developing diabetes, hypertension, or both, or at least delay the onset of both diseases.

Alternative Therapies for Diabetes and Hypertension

Over 5 million American have both diabetes and high blood pressure. In May of 2000, the National Institutes of Health published an advisory for people who have both hypertension and diabetes. The NIH recommends that physicians be aggressive in their efforts to lower the blood pressure of patients affected by both diseases, since diabetes and hypertension are independent risk factors for cardiovascular disease (CVD). The coexistence of these conditions sets a blood pressure goal as 135/80 mm Hg, slightly lower than the goal for those who have only one or neither disease.

The NIH is also exploring alternative therapies to manage diabetes. These alternative therapies include acupuncture, biofeedback, guided imagery, and vitamin and mineral supplementation. The success of some alternative treatments can be hard to measure. Many alternative treatments remain either untested or unproven through traditional scientific studies.

Here are some of the alternative therapies that seem to show promise for diabetics. Notice that the same therapies are used in the treatment of high blood pressure.

Acupuncture is a procedure in which a practitioner inserts needles into designated points on the skin. Some Western scientists believe that acupuncture triggers the release of the body's natural painkillers. Acupuncture has been shown to offer relief from chronic pain. Acupuncture is sometimes used to relieve the painful nerve damage of diabetes. For more about acupuncture, see Chapter 28.

Biofeedback is a technique that helps a person become more aware of and learn to deal with the body's automatic response internal messages and pain. This alternative therapy emphasizes relaxation and stress-reduction techniques. For more about biofeedback in the treatment of hypertension and diabetes, see Chapter 27.

Guided imagery is a relaxation technique that some professionals who use biofeedback do. With guided imagery, a person thinks of peaceful mental images, such as ocean waves. A person may also include images of controlling or curing a chronic disease, such as hypertension or diabetes. People using this technique believe their conditions can be eased with these positive images. For more information about relaxation techniques, see Chapter 26.

Magnesium supplements in the treatment both of hypertension and diabetes have been studied for decades Studies suggest that a deficiency in magnesium may worsen the blood sugar control in diabetes; the role of magnesium, working in conjunction with calcium and potassium, in regulating blood pressure has been accepted. The level of magnesium in the blood is regulated by the kidneys. For more about magnesium supplements in the treatment of hypertension, see Chapter 18.

Chromium is needed to make glucose tolerance factor, which helps insulin improve its action. It is now being studied and debated by many authorities, but no recommendations for chromium supplements yet exist.

Note: to learn more about alternative therapies for diabetes and high blood pressure treatment, contact the National Institutes of Health's Office of Alternative Medicines Clearinghouse at 888-644-6226, or visit www.niddk.nih.gov.

CHAPTER 16

Hypertension: A Risk Factor for Stroke

Stroke is the third leading killer in the United States. Each year, more than half a million Americans have a stroke, with more than a hundred thousand deaths. The most common cause of adult disability, a stroke, can be devastating and can steal your independence.

Warning Signs of a Stroke

Your body sends you warnings when your brain does not receive enough oxygen. These are the warning signs of a stroke. If you have one or more of these symptoms it is an emergency and you should call a doctor or 911 right away!

- Sudden weakness or numbness of the face, arm, or leg.
- Sudden dimness or loss of vision, particularly in one eye.
- Sudden severe headache with no known cause.
- Unexplained dizziness, unsteadiness, or sudden falls, especially when combined with other signs.
- Other danger signs include double vision, drowsiness, and nausea or vomiting.

Sometimes the warning signs may last only a few moments and then disappear. These short episodes, known as transient ischemic attacks (TIAs), point to an underlying serious condition and indicate the necessity of seeking medical help. Don't ignore them. The faster you get treatment, the better the outcome will be.

> ## Early HBP Treatment for Good Thinking
>
> A study at the University of Kansas reveals that treating high blood pressure in midlife helps prevent strokes and senility later. Researchers found that even moderately high blood pressure is linked to faster aging of the brain. Smoking, drinking, and diabetes had similar, but smaller, risks. The scientists concluded that early high blood pressure treatment can prevent the small strokes that may cause dementia.

STROKE RISK FACTORS—AND HOW TO CONTROL THEM

A risk factor is a physical condition or lifestyle habit that significantly correlates with a particular disease. Having a risk factor for stroke doesn't mean you'll have a stroke, and not having any of the risk factors doesn't mean you'll avoid having a stroke. However, your risk of a stroke grows as the number of risk factors increases. The best way to prevent a stroke is to eliminate as many risk factors as possible, especially since there are risk factors that can't be controlled, such as age, sex, race, diabetes mellitus, and a prior stroke.

Age is certainly a factor. The older a person is, the greater the stroke risk. Men are more likely to have a stroke, and those with diabetes are at still higher risk. About 10 percent of strokes are preceded by "temporary strokes" (transient ischemic attacks, TIAs). These can occur days, weeks, or even months before a major stroke. Medical treatment can address some factors: high blood pressure, heart disease, the treatment of a TIA. High blood pressure, which is controllable, and which can be controlled through a healthy lifestyle and medication, is by far one of the most potent risk factors for stroke.

LOWERING YOUR RISK

You can also reduce your risk factors by changing your lifestyle. You can lower your cholesterol level, stop smoking, and avoid high alcohol intake. Cigarette smoking has been linked to the buildup of fatty substances in the carotid artery, the main neck artery supplying blood to the brain. Blockage of this artery is the leading cause of stroke in Americans. Nicotine also raises blood pressure. Carbon monoxide from smoking reduces the

> ## *Nighttime Blood Pressure Is an Important Risk Indicator*
>
> Normally, blood pressure lowers at night during sleep. However, Japanese researchers have found that hypertensive people who show no dip in systolic pressure while sleeping seem to be most at risk for stroke. Scientists at the Kyoto Red Cross Hospital divided patients into groups, from those who showed no symptoms of stroke or development of new brain lesions to patients who had more extensive cerebrovascular disease. The results showed that patients with no symptoms had on average a nighttime systolic blood pressure that was 10 points lower than their daytime blood pressure. In patients with the most severe damage, the dip was minuscule, averaging less than 4 points lower.

amount of oxygen the blood can carry to the brain. Cigarette smoke also makes blood thicker and more likely to clot.

Diagnosis and Treatment

If you are in a high-risk group, or have any warning signs, you should be treated by your family doctor or a neurologist. Only a physician can evaluate the problem. An early diagnosis is made by evaluating symptoms, reviewing medical history, and performing several tests. Tests that may be given include an electrocardiogram and an electroencephalogram (a test that measures nerve cell activity in the brain), as well as other tests and advanced brain scanning.

Treatment begins as soon as the stroke is diagnosed—the speedier the treatment is started, the better. Anticoagulants may be prescribed to prevent blood clots from becoming larger; or, in the case of hemorrhagic stroke, drugs to lower blood pressure may be prescribed. Some studies have indicted that even at low dosage, the blood-thinning properties of aspirin can lower the risk of a second stroke by 25 to 50 percent.

The good news is that a better understanding of the causes of stroke has helped Americans make lifestyle changes that have cut the stroke death rate nearly in half in the last two decades. The scientists at the National Institute of Neurological Disorders and Stroke (NIH Neurological Institute, P.O. Box 5801, Bethesda, MD 20824; 800-352-9424) have stated that with con-tinued attention to reducing the risks of stroke and by using currently available therapies while developing new ones, Americans should be able to prevent about 80 percent of all strokes in the new century.

CHAPTER 17

Working Together: The Pump and the Hose

Besides straining the kidneys and arteries, high blood pressure strains the heart. Although the heart pumps out only two or three ounces of blood with each contraction, it does this 60 to 80 times a minute when at rest, or more than 100,000 times a day, pumping roughly 2,000 gallons of blood. This is an astonishing volume for an organ about the size of two clenched fists and weighing from 11 to 16 ounces in adults (though it becomes larger and heavier with age).

Cardiovascular disease (CVD), the leading cause of death in the United States, killed almost a million people in 1995—41.5 percent of all deaths. It is estimated that almost 60 million people have one or more types of CVD, which includes high blood pressure.

Heart Failure

Heart failure is exactly what the words describe: The heart fails to pump the blood through the arteries and veins. The heart pumps blood against resistance. When the resistance is low, the heart uses less energy. When there is greater resistance, the heart must work harder to pump blood.

At first, the heart will adjust to this resistance by increasing its size. This is called hypertrophy. Think about weight lifters you see at the Olympic games or on television advertisements for muscle-building machines. How do they get their muscles so large? Weight lifters add small amounts of weights periodically when they exercise. This encourages the muscles to thicken. The heart thickens in a similar way. When this happens, the heart appears larger, but basically only the muscle walls enlarge, not the interior chambers. Eventually, the heart can no longer increase its ability to pump and it will fail.

Any resistance that the blood flow meets on its way through the arteries will add to the heart's labor, making it pump harder to get blood to every organ and tissue in the body. The extra effort results in a rise in blood pressure. Heart health and blood pressure are linked; one seriously affects the other.

WHO IS AT RISK?

As with many other risk factors, some can be changed and some cannot. Although these factors increase the risk of coronary heart disease, they do not describe all the causes. Even with none of these factors you still might develop the disease.

Controllable Risk Factors	Uncontrollable Risk Factors
High blood pressure	Age
High blood cholesterol	Family history
Smoking	
Obesity	
Physical inactivity	
Diabetes	
Stress (see Chapter 25)	

Note: Do you notice that the risk factors for heart disease are the same as those for hypertension? When you lower your blood pressure through any of these controllable factors your heart as well as your arteries will thank you!

WARNING SIGNALS OF HEART ATTACK

When you suffer a heart attack, every second counts. Don't wait to get help. Be sure you know these signs because they are important to your life:

- Uncomfortable pressure, fullness, squeezing, or pain in the center of the chest lasting more than a few minutes
- Pain that has spread to the shoulders, neck, or arms

♦ Chest discomfort with light-headedness, fainting, sweating, nausea, or shortness of breath

When the heart muscle doesn't get enough oxygen-carrying blood, it begins to die. This causes the unpleasant and painful reactions of heart attack.

Heart-Smart Test

Below is a test developed by the National Heart, Lung, and Blood Institute. Answer true or false to the following questions to test your knowledge of the interrelationship between heart disease and hypertension. Here is a clue: All the answers are also related to controlling high blood pressure. (This is an informal questionnaire, so just jot down your answers on a piece of paper.) Check the answers and you'll see the links between the two health problems.

1. The risk factors for heart disease that you can do something about are: high blood pressure, high blood cholesterol, smoking, obesity, and physical inactivity.

2. A stroke is often the first symptom of high blood pressure, and a heart attack is often the first symptom of high blood cholesterol.

3. A blood pressure greater than or equal to 140/90 mm Hg is generally considered high.

4. High blood pressure affects the same number of people in all ethnic groups.

5. The best ways to treat and control high blood pressure are to control your weight, exercise, eat less salt (sodium), restrict your intake of alcohol, stop smoking, and take medicine if it is prescribed by your doctor.

6. A blood cholesterol level of 240 mg/dl is desirable for adults.

7. The most effective dietary way to lower your blood cholesterol is to eat foods low in cholesterol.

8. Lowering blood cholesterol levels can help people who have already had a heart attack.

9. Only children from families at high risk of heart disease need to have their blood cholesterol levels checked.

10. Smoking is a risk factor for four of the five leading causes of death, including heart attack, stroke, hypertension, and cancer.

11. If you have had a heart attack, stop smoking. It can help reduce your chances of having a second attack.

12. Someone who has smoked for thirty or more years will probably not be able to quit smoking.

13. The best way to lose weight is to increase physical activity and eat fewer calories.

14. Heart disease is the leading killer of men and women in the United States.

Here are the answers:

1—True: High blood pressure, high blood cholesterol, and smoking are the three most important risk factors for heart disease. On average each one doubles your chance of developing heart disease. That means a person who has all three of these risk factors is eight times more likely to develop heart disease than someone who has none.

Obesity increases the likelihood of developing high blood pressure and high blood cholesterol; both increase your risk for heart disease. Physical inactivity increases your risk of heart attack. Regular exercise and good nutrition are essential to reducing high blood pressure and high blood cholesterol. Overweight people who exercise are also more likely to cut down or stop smoking.

2—True: A person with high blood pressure may feel fine and look great, as there is often no sign that anything is wrong until a stroke or heart attack occurs. To find out if you have high blood pressure or high blood cholesterol, you should be tested by a physician or other health professional.

3—True: A blood pressure of 140/90 mm Hg or greater is generally classified as high blood pressure. However, blood pressures that fall below 140/90 mm Hg can sometimes be a problem. If the diastolic pressure, the second or lower number, is between 85 and 89, a person is at increased risk for heart disease or stroke and should have his or her blood pressure checked at least once a year by a health professional. The higher your blood pressure, the greater your risk of developing heart disease or stroke. Controlling high blood pressure reduces your risk.

> ## Morning Warning
>
> As we have seen, blood pressure is at its lowest at night about 3:00 A.M., when you are asleep. It rises rapidly between 6:00 A.M. and noon—just as you rush to start your stressful day. These hours are also the time when heart attacks, strokes, and fatal heart failures most often occur. Do you think it may be best to start your day slowly?

4—False: High blood pressure is more common in African-Americans than in white Americans. It affects 29 out of every 100 black adults, compared with 26 out of every 100 white adults. Also, with aging, high blood pressure is generally more severe among African-Americans than among whites, and therefore causes more strokes, heart disease, and kidney failure.

5—True: Recent studies show that lifestyle changes can help keep blood pressure normal even into advanced age and are important in treating and preventing high blood pressure. It is extremely important to check your blood pressure and make sure it stays under control.

6—False: A total cholesterol level of 200 mg/dl is good. Levels above that are high and increase your risk of heart disease. If your cholesterol level is high, your doctor will want to check your levels of LDL (the bad cholesterol) and HDL cholesterol (the good cholesterol). A high level of LDL cholesterol increases your risk of heart disease, as does a low level of HDL cholesterol.

A cholesterol level of between 200 and 239 mg/dl is considered borderline high and usually increases your risk of heart disease. If your cholesterol is borderline high, you should speak to your doctor to see if additional cholesterol tests are needed. All adults twenty years of age or older should have their blood cholesterol level checked at least once every five years.

7—False: Reducing the amount of cholesterol in your diet is important; however, eating foods low in saturated fat is the most effective way to lower blood cholesterol levels, along with eating less total fat and cholesterol.

8—True: People who have had one heart attack are at much higher risk for a second heart attack. Reducing blood cholesterol levels can greatly slow down (and, in some people, even reverse) the buildup of cholesterol

---

Rats Get Hypertension, Too

In 1990 experimental prevention of hypertension and related cardiovascular disease was studied in laboratory rats. The experiments show that salt reduction was not enough to lower blood pressure. Increased intakes of potassium, calcium, magnesium, protein, and omega-3 fatty acids and dietary fiber did, however, prove effective. These studies indicate the importance of nonpharmacological dietary prevention of cardiovascular disease.

---

and fat in the walls of the coronary arteries and significantly reduce the chances of a second heart attack.

9—True: Children from high-risk families, in which a parent has high blood cholesterol (240 mg/dl or above) or in which a parent or grandparent has had heart disease or high blood pressure at an early age, should have their cholesterol levels tested. If a child from such a family has high cholesterol, it should be lowered under medical supervision, primarily with diet, to reduce the risk of developing heart disease and high blood pressure as an adult. All children, whether or not from high-risk families, can best reduce the risk of adult heart disease by following a low-saturated-fat, low-cholesterol eating pattern.

10—True: Heavy smokers are two to four times more likely to have a heart attack than nonsmokers. Smoking also affects blood pressure and increases your chance of stroke. The heart attack death rate among all smokers is 70 percent greater than that of nonsmokers. Older male smokers are also nearly twice as likely to die from stroke than older men who do not smoke, and these odds are nearly as high for older female smokers. The risk of dying of lung cancer is twenty-two times higher for male smokers than male nonsmokers, and twelve times higher for female smokers than female nonsmokers. Finally, 80 percent of all deaths from emphysema and bronchitis are due to smoking.

11—True: Even if you have already had a heart attack, you can reduce your chances of having a second attack if you quit smoking. One year after quitting, ex-smokers cut their risk of heart attack by about half or more. Eventually, the risk will return to normal in healthy ex-smokers. Ex-smokers also reduce their risk of stroke and cancer, show improved

Heart-Loving Vegetables

Vitamins C and E and beta-carotene have been identified as showing potential to fight against coronary heart disease. Here are some foods that should be part of your diet:

Beta-carotene: carrots, pumpkins, spinach, squash, sweet potatoes

Vitamin C: berries, broccoli, cantaloupe, citrus fruits, peppers (red and green)

Vitamin E: kale, spinach, sunflower seeds, turnip greens, whole grains

blood flow and lung function, and avoid many respiratory diseases. Quitting also helps relieve smoking-related symptoms like shortness of breath, coughing, and chest pain.

12—False: Older smokers are actually more likely to succeed at quitting smoking than younger smokers. Many quit to avoid further health problems and take control of their lives.

13—True: Weight control is a question of balance. You get calories from the food you eat. You burn off calories by exercising. Cutting down on calories, especially calories from fat, is the key to losing weight. Combining this with a regular physical activity, like walking, cycling, jogging, or swimming, can help in losing weight and in maintaining weight loss.

A steady weight loss of one-half to one pound a week is safe for most adults, and the weight is more likely to stay off over the long run. Losing weight, if you are overweight, may also help reduce your blood pressure and lower your LDL cholesterol. Being physically active and eating fewer calories will also help you prevent the weight gain many experience when quitting smoking.

Wash Out the Smoke

When you quit smoking, drink a lot of water or other watery liquids. Water can counter some of the nicotine cravings. Water acts as a natural diuretic. Many fresh vegetables also have a slightly diuretic effect.

14—True: Coronary heart disease is the number one killer in the United States. High blood pressure affects over 50 million people in the United States. They are two related diseases, and you can fight both at the same time. It will double your results!

For more information write for a magazine-style booklet, *Hearts and Arteries,* from the National Heart, Lung, and Blood Institute, Information Center, P.O. Box 30105, Bethesda, MD 20824-0105.

CHAPTER 18

Potassium, Calcium, and Magnesium and High Blood Pressure

The mineral elements sodium, potassium, calcium, and magnesium are central in the normal regulation of blood pressure while enhancing arterial health. Potassium and especially calcium also regulate the body's fluid balance and influence blood flow.

Minerals Make a Difference

In 1991, researchers in Finland published their findings that certain levels of these mineral elements in diets may protect people against developing hypertension. People with a high consumption of potassium, and possibly magnesium, don't seem to develop arterial hypertension, and there is less evidence of a rise of blood pressure with age.

In hypertensive people treated with antihypertensive drugs, restricting dietary sodium while supplementing their diet with calcium, potassium, and magnesium enhances the therapeutic effect of antihypertensive medications. The supplements can also reduce the dosage needed to control HBP. Calcium and potassium also seem to lessen the adverse side effects of antihypertensive drugs.

The Importance of Potassium

Potassium is a chemical component with many properties similar to those of sodium. However, potassium is a chemical within the body cells; sodium is a major chemical in the fluid between and around the cells. The two are interrelated in the complex mechanisms of body functioning.

A May 1999 Johns Hopkins University study clarified the link. Researchers gave participants about 3,000 milligrams of potassium, and these supplements lowered systolic blood pressure by 3.1 points and diastolic pressure by 2.0 points. Potassium proved more helpful in people with severe high blood pressure and those who ate high-salt diets.

HOW MUCH POTASSIUM?

There is no recommended dietary allowance (RDA) for potassium. The average intake is between 2,000 and 3,500 milligrams a day, and comes from either food or supplements. The recent DASH diet recommends 4,700 milligrams of potassium a day. Daily consumption of 2,000 to 6,000 milligrams of potassium, however, is within the safe range for the average person. Negative side effects are rare, and mostly minor, such as belching and flatulence.

Since small amounts of potassium most likely play a role in lowering high blood pressure, eating foods that are high in potassium is a good idea for people with hypertension or those at risk. I follow my own advice to patients and drink my orange juice and eat a banana or apple for a snack. It is a perfect midday snack for me. We also microwave or steam all our vegetables to preserve their potassium content.

Nature has put potassium in so many foods that few people who eat a balanced diet are deficient in it. It is so well controlled by the body—excreted with such ease—that slightly excessive intake has no ill effects on a healthy person.

WHEN IS POTASSIUM NEEDED, AND WHEN IS IT DANGEROUS?

Some people lose potassium because they take antihypertensive diuretics to remove sodium from the body. Others lose it as a result of diarrhea or vomiting. To replace potassium and keep the body's chemicals in balance, nutritionists often recommend that these patients eat bananas and potatoes. Some people may also require potassium tablets to make up for the deficiency.

Potassium alert: Too much potassium in the blood is called hyperkalemia, and can be serious, even life-threatening. In kidney disease, where potassium is not adequately excreted, excess potassium can cause serious

Potassium-Rich Foods (in milligrams)

Potato (1 medium)	755
Avocado (½ medium)	604
Banana (1 medium)	550
Nonfat milk (1 cup)	308
Red beans (⅔ cup, cooked)	340
Orange (1 medium)	300
Cantaloupe (¼ melon)	251
Dates (½ cup)	380

complications. In such people, dietary control of potassium is necessary. In rare cases, excess potassium can lead to kidney failure. Those who have diabetes mellitus have a defect in the kidney's ability to regulate potassium levels.

There are also several medications that can cause potassium buildup, including aspirin and ibuprofen, so checking with your physician before taking such medications is a must. Because of this, some experts feel that the potassium content of common foods should be listed along with the sodium content in all nutrition labels.

POTASSIUM IN FOODS

The U.S. Department of Agriculture recommends catfish, cod, flounder, trout, and sardines as good sources of potassium. Lean pork, beef, and veal also provide potassium. Eating a diet high in fruits and vegetables almost assures you of getting enough of the mineral. Microwave or steam all your vegetables, which will preserve the potassium. A bonus of a potassium-rich diet is that it is usually very high in fiber, another important part of a healthy diet.

Calcium's Contribution

One of the most abundant elements on earth, calcium is found in bones, shells, and limestone. It is necessary for both plant and animal life. The diets of all mammals are rich in calcium. The diet of the stone age human is estimated to have contained three to five times the calcium intake of the present-day adult American's diet.

The human body contains more calcium than any other of the essential minerals. (An essential mineral is one that the body requires in amounts greater than 100 milligrams daily.) People have about two and a half pounds of this mineral in their body, most of it in their bones. Since this essential nutrient cannot be manufactured in the body, we need a daily supply for our teeth and bones. It plays an important role in blood clotting, too. Calcium is essential to our nervous system and to the normal functioning of body cells.

Although our bodies contain mechanisms by which we can adjust to temporary environmental shortages, chronic calcium depletion has a number of dire health consequences, including bone fragility, colon cancer, and high blood pressure. Research and evidence suggest that adequate calcium may protect against salt-sensitive and pregnancy-associated hypertension.

WHERE TO GET CALCIUM?

The chief sources of calcium are milk and milk products, dark green vegetables, and shellfish. Many foods contain some calcium, but few foods contain sufficient amounts of calcium to fulfill your body's daily needs. Additionally your body may not be able to absorb all the calcium you take in from foods and from supplements.

Since so much of our calcium comes from dairy products, researchers say that eliminating dairy products from your diet can result in a calcium deficiency. These claims, while interesting, are not convincing, since many cultures lack dairy calcium in their native cuisines.

HOW MUCH CALCIUM IS NEEDED?

Nutritionists at the Department of Agriculture set the recommended daily allowance for calcium at about 800 mg, although 1,000 mg has been recommended for most people. Other government experts recommend that adults under age fifty should aim for 1,000 mg daily, while people over fifty should try for 1,200 mg daily. Daily this means two to three cups of milk, which will provide 600 to 900 mg of calcium. The lactose in milk and milk products also enhances calcium absorption.

Dairy products are by far America's favorite source of calcium. Most of

> ### *Raw Is Best for Calcium*
>
> Cooking diminishes the calcium content of vegetables. For example, 3½ oz of cooked kale contain 134 mg of calcium as opposed to 179 mg raw; cooked turnip greens have 184 mg of calcium but 246 mg raw. Fruits usually have little or no calcium.

us get 75 percent of our daily requirements from dairy products, a scant 7 percent from meat, fish, and poultry and from vegetables, and 11 percent from cereals and other foods.

Do you like broccoli? You would have to eat two cups of broccoli to get the same amount of calcium contained in one cup of milk. But there is a downside: A glass of whole milk has as much saturated fat as three strips of bacon, and saturated fats increase your chances of developing clogged arteries. When you select your calcium source, look for low-fat milk. Skim milk and 1 percent low-fat milk are widely available; they are the right choice for anyone with HBP.

By itself, corn is not a significant source of calcium. However, cornmeal can be made by soaking corn in a lime solution of calcium oxide to remove its tough outer coating. When the corn is washed, drained, and ground some of the calcium remains. One corn tortilla contains about 40 mg of calcium. By comparison, eight ounces of milk contain about 300 mg.

CALCIUM STUDIES: THE JURY IS STILL OUT

Too little calcium in the diet may be a little recognized factor contributing to high blood pressure, according to a study at Oregon Health Sciences University several years ago. The researchers found that the amounts of milk and nondairy products containing calcium were present in equal quantities in hypertensives and in those who were not hypertensive, but that those in the study with high blood pressure consumed fewer dairy products other than milk than did people with normal blood pressure.

Ironically, many researchers believe that in certain circumstances calcium may cause hypertension. They believe that the passage of calcium into and out of cells brings about the degree of tightness that determines the blood pressure within our arteries. When there is a shortage of calcium, relaxation of the artery walls is insufficient to allow blood to flow freely, and the result is hypertension. The findings are not altogether convinc-

Other Calcium Sources

Dairy products are the best sources of calcium. Here are some other good sources. For about 300–400 milligrams of calcium, eat:

Sardines with bones (oily sardines are also high in omega-3 fatty acids)

Tofu processed with calcium (read label)

Café latte (so chic and tastes good too)

Salmon, canned with bones (you need a big serving)

Collard, kale, or other dark greens (steamed or microwaved)

Fortified orange juice (read the label)

Almonds (a handful, not salted)

Frozen yogurt (nonfat)

Clams or shrimp (a large serving)

Soups, creamed (high in fat)

ing, but they have attracted the interest of many people in the medical community.

In the early 1990s an enthusiastic dairy industry trumpeted that an adequate dietary intake of calcium may reduce the risk of high blood pressure. They issued a report citing hundreds of studies supporting this claim. However, according to many experts, the evidence isn't conclusive. While many studies do show that low levels of calcium correlate with high blood pressure, there's no solid proof that adding calcium to the diet can prevent or control high blood pressure. However, there are many other reasons to get enough calcium: Adequate dietary calcium is the best defense against osteoporosis.

VITAMIN D AND CALCIUM

Your body cannot absorb calcium if you're deficient in vitamin D, or if you don't get enough sunlight. Even though your body can produce vitamin D when you're exposed to sunlight, people who live in cloudy or smoggy climates, as well as office workers who are indoors all the time, benefit from vitamin D supplements. Your body also is less efficient in manufacturing vitamin D as you get older. The recommended dietary allowance for vitamin D is 400 international units, the amount in one quart of milk. Many calcium supplements are also fortified with vitamin D.

Too much vitamin D can cause problems: Large doses might cause nausea, weakness, headache, digestive problems, and kidney and heart damage. Excess vitamin D has also been linked with calcification of soft issue, which is the depositing of calcium into organ tissues.

CALCIUM LOSS

In older people, a loss of calcium causes the bones to weaken and soften, a condition called osteoporosis; this is particularly prevalent in post-menopausal women. Long periods of bed rest will also cause loss of calcium from the bones. People who have broken a hip and cannot move around may find it difficult to regain easy use of their limbs as a result of calcium loss. Here are other calcium enemies:

- High alcohol consumption interferes with calcium absorption.

- Coffee also contributes to calcium deficiency. Some studies show that older women who consume several cups of coffee a day have a higher chance of having osteoporosis than those who don't. Many experts believe that the diuretic property of coffee is partly to blame.

- Certain prescription drugs can actively lower the body's calcium level. Discuss this with your doctor.

- Smoking is thought to be linked with the loss of calcium from the bones.

- Fiber, bran in particular, in excessive amounts has been linked with preventing calcium absorption.

CALCIUM SUPPLEMENTS

If your diet is not high in dairy foods, you may need to take calcium supplements. The National Institutes of Health recommend taking no more than 500 milligrams in supplements. Most supplements should be taken between meals; however, the decision to take the supplements with or between meals may depend on the type of supplement taken. Dietary supplements include:

Calcium carbonate (the most common type of calcium supplement) is best absorbed when it is taken with foods, especially acidic foods such as citrus juice or fruit. Calcium carbonate is about 40 percent calcium. Note:

Calcium carbonate combined with vitamins D and K is now available in chewy candies, and each candy is only 20 calories a candy.

Calcium citrate is best absorbed on an empty stomach. The citrate form does not require gastric acid for absorption. It is the preferred supplement for those who lack gastric acid or those who are taking medications that block gastric acid production.

Calcium phosphate contains about 20 percent calcium.

Calcium lactate is slightly more easily absorbed than other supplements. Calcium is about 18 percent calcium.

Tums provides about 250 mg of calcium per tablet.

WHEN AND HOW OF CALCIUM SUPPLEMENTS

There is no consensus on how to take supplements: The type and amount of calcium you take as a supplement should be based on your medical history and your average dietary intake of calcium. However, most nutritionists agree supplements should be taken in small amounts of less than 500 mg, throughout the day. If you are also taking an iron supplement, don't take calcium at the same time you take the iron, since the iron could block calcium absorption. Remember your potassium and vitamin D intake when you take calcium supplements. Both regulate acid levels in your blood. Avoid supplemental calcium from such sources as dolomite, oyster shell, and bonemeal, which may be contaminated with toxic metals.

TOO MUCH CALCIUM

Large amounts of calcium (2,500 mg per day) may not cause problems for healthy people, but for people with kidney disease, a large intake of calcium can produce serious complications. Some people develop kidney stones when they have an excessive amount of calcium. We do not know why this occurs in some people and not in others.

Kidney stones are a fairly common problem. They often start with severe pain, called renal colic; at times the condition can be painless. Since stones can destroy the kidney, once they are discovered they can require hospital care and surgery. However, a new technique in which the kidney stone is pulverized with sound waves seems to work wonders—with no surgery.

Can you prevent calcium buildup by reducing your intake of foods that are high in calcium? Not a good idea! Although calcium is one of several elements that make up plaque, a substance that contributes to atherosclerosis, calcium in your food has no effect on the buildup of calcium in blood vessels. It is thought that calcification results from plaque buildup, rather than causing it.

The Significance of Magnesium

Magnesium is a mineral that forms part of your bones. It has been linked with bone mineral density and the transmission of nerve impulses to muscles. In conjunction with calcium and potassium, magnesium is active in regulating blood pressure. Researchers who worked with the Honolulu heart program studied the diets of healthy older people and found that people with the highest magnesium intake had the lowest blood pressure. The level of magnesium in the blood is regulated by the kidneys. Researchers at the medical university in Kobe, Japan, studied the relationship between magnesium and blood pressure. For one month, they gave patients with mild hypertension 600 milligrams of magnesium a day. The patients' pressure went down.

HOW MUCH MAGNESIUM IS NEEDED?

We usually absorb the magnesium we need from food. If you eat about three servings of vegetables and grains a day and have legumes twice a week, you are probably getting enough magnesium from your food. However, fast food diets are not high in magnesium. Here is a small chart listing some magnesium-rich foods.

Eat Nuts		
Almonds	1 oz	86 mg
Pumpkin seeds	1 oz	150 mg
Soybean nuts	4 oz	195 mg
Peanut butter	2 oz	50 mg

Bran cereals, peanut butter, seeds, beans, and green vegetables are high in magnesium. If you like baked potatoes (high in potassium), eat the skin, too, and you'll be getting good quantities of this mineral. Magnesium also occurs in drinking water (except soft water).

Milk of magnesia, a laxative, provides about 1,000 mg in just two table-spoons. We need between 300 and 450 mg of magnesium daily, but too much can be dangerous: Drowsiness, lethargy, sweating, and slurred speech are signs of an overdose.

Potassium, calcium, and magnesium have been studied and found to be important in controlling hypertension. In reading through this section, you probably noticed a pattern: milk, vegetables, beans, and nuts are important in your diet. The recent advent of "nutriceutical" foods (orange juice supplemented with calcium, for example) constitutes an important advance in our diets.

PART III

Your Style of Living

You may not have to depend on medicines if you learn some new habits and discard a few old ones. Mark Twain once said, "Habit is habit, and not to be flung out of the window by anyone, but coaxed downstairs a step at a time." Which habits should be coaxed downstairs?

Selecting foods that are good for you, reducing alcohol intake and eliminating smoking, exercising and becoming more active, learning to identify and avoid stress, and learning how to replace anxiety with calm may take some practice, but such habits will bring happiness and peace into your life—as well as lower your blood pressure.

CHAPTER 19

Smoke Gets in Your Blood

S moking is nothing less than taking a toxic substance into the body. Cigarette smoking harms many body functions and adversely affects your blood pressure.

Clear Evidence of Smoking's Harm

We have known for many years that smoking can produce a significant rise in the pulse rate as well as a rise in both systolic and diastolic blood pressure. More than a quarter century ago, Dr. Philip E. Cryer of Washington University School of Medicine in St. Louis, Missouri, writing in *The New England Journal of Medicine,* said, "Within 2.5 minutes after a person started to smoke there was a rise in the pulse rate; systolic and diastolic pressure increased by a total of about 12 points. There was no rise in pressure and pulse rate in a control group given placebo cigarettes."

There have been many other studies too: Some show a link between hypertension and smoking, some show that smoking increases the risk of heart and blood vessel diseases. This applies as well to filtered cigarettes and to "passive smoking" (inhaling the smoke when near a person who smokes). Smoking poses risks for a wide range of diseases. One study reported that smokers have blood pressure up to 10 points higher than nonsmokers. The problems brought on by every puff have become more and more evident. Smoking has also become socially unacceptable in almost all public buildings, public transportation, and offices.

Two decades ago, about 30 percent of Americans smoked cigarettes.

Smoking Contaminants

When you smoke, you expose yourself to some 4,000 chemicals. Every time you inhale you breathe in: Acetaldehyde acetone, ammonia, argon, cadmium, carbon dioxide, DDT, hydrogen sulfide, hydrogen cyanide, lead, methane, nickel, nicotine, phenol, and other gases. This affects almost every vessel in your body. Cigarette smoke constricts your blood vessels, which makes your heart work harder to force blood through your arteries and veins.

Now fewer than 25 percent of us smoke. Many of today's smokers are young people, with a high percentage of young women, who believe smoking will help them lose weight and quitting will lead to weight gain. Among these people are a large number who would like to stop but feel they can't.

Smoking affects almost every vessel in your body. Cosmetic surgeons have noticed that nonsmokers seem to heal more rapidly and have better outcomes than heavy smokers. Nicotine-laced smoke also weakens the ability of some prescribed hypertension medications and other medications to do their job. Smoking increases any tendency to develop brain hemorrhages and is implicated in the rare, but severe, kind of high blood pressure known as malignant hypertension. Note: Cigars, no matter how expensive they are or elegant they look, are as harmful as cigarettes. Pipe smoking is also harmful.

Why You Should Quit Now

If you stopped today, you would see some immediate benefits: Your body begins to heal from the effects of nicotine within twelve hours after your last cigarette or cigar. You'll avoid bad breath, you'll feel better, cough less, have fewer stomach problems, less carbon monoxide in your blood—and more money.

The long-term benefits you would enjoy include a decline in the risk of heart disease within a year; after ten years heart attack risk factors will be normal for age and weight. Lung cancer risk declines after two years of not smoking; after twelve years of not smoking, your mortality rate will be the same as someone who never smoked.

If you want to stop, what are the chances that you will be successful? According to government studies, smokers who want to stop will do so if they are sufficiently motivated and they receive professional help. One of the most effective initial aids in getting people to stop smoking is their physician's suggestion that they stop.

WHEN YOU'RE READY

Programs to help you quit are offered by the following groups, as well as many local hospitals and health centers:

Agency for Health Care Policy and Research, 800-358-9295,
http://www.ahcpr.gov/

American Heart Association, 800-AHA-USA1 (800-242-8721),
http://www.americanheart.org

American Cancer Society, 800-ACS-2345 (800-227-2345),
http://www.lungusa.org/

American Lung Association, 800-LUNG-USA (800-586-4872),
http://www.lungusa.org/

Office of Smoking and Health, Centers for Disease Control and
Prevention, 800-CDC-1311 (800-232-1311),
http://www.cdc.gov/tobacco/

QUITTING ISN'T EASY

Habitual smoking is an addiction to nicotine. Nicotine stimulates the brain's electrical activity, resulting in a sense of intensified satisfaction. Nicotine also acts on "binding sites" in the brain and throughout the body. It gets into the brain faster and more easily than many other drugs, penetrating the blood-brain barrier as quickly as illegal drugs such as heroin.

In 1988, a Surgeon General's report conclusively demonstrated that "cigarettes and other forms of tobacco are just as addicting as illegal drugs." Many smokers who find it hard to quit can testify to nicotine's power. Those who are physically dependent undergo the discomfort of withdrawal if they stop smoking. But if you don't succeed at first, keep trying. Don't be discouraged if it takes several tries.

> ## Smokeless Poison
>
> Smokeless tobacco (chewing tobacco) contains large amounts of sodium to enhance flavor and help your body absorb the nicotine. It has no place in any kind of blood-pressure-lowering program. Young men might think it is macho to chew, but if you turn to Chapter 24, you'll learn about the link between nicotine-constricted blood vessels and impotence. Another nasty outcome of chewing tobacco is an increased risk of mouth cancer.

THE STRESS AND SMOKE CYCLE

A study published in the October 1999 issue of *American Psychologist* examined one of tobacco's paradoxes. Smokers say that lighting up provides a sense of relief and well-being. However, many smokers report tension and stress between cigarettes. One explanation may be that people with high levels of stress are drawn to smoking. More likely, smokers are suffering the whipsaw effect of a habit/addiction. According to Dr. Andy Parrott, a psychologist in London, "The regular smoker needs nicotine to maintain normal moods and suffers from unpleasant feelings of irritability between cigarettes when his or her plasma nicotine levels are falling."

Although many smokers can control their nicotine intake by shortening the extent and frequency of the inhalation of smoke, quitting cold turkey is easier for most than a gradual reduction in the number of cigarettes smoked. The withdrawal symptoms also subside more rapidly when the cutoff is sudden. The withdrawal symptoms vary with the individual.

THE DOCTOR TAKES HIS OWN ADVICE

I don't believe all smokers are as nicotine-dependent as some studies would suggest. Just as there are social drinkers who can stop after one or two drinks, there are some smokers for whom smoking is less compelling. My own response to smoking was never very intense. I found quitting relatively simple, perhaps because I know what nicotine can do to anyone's total health.

As a first step, try to go it alone. Although this method for giving up smoking seems the least complicated and the easiest, it may actually prove most difficult. However, start out with the determination that you are going to have sufficient willpower to make a dead stop. Throw your cigarettes and your habit into the garbage. This was the method I used about ten years ago. I made up my mind to stop, and I did, although it was not always easy.

I remember only one extremely difficult situation. It was when I had to give a patient some bad news. As I sat at the bedside of a very young man and started to tell him about the severity of his illness, he reached into the bedside table drawer and took out a fresh pack of cigarettes, the same brand I enjoyed smoking. He opened the pack and offered me one. I reached for the cigarette but then got control of myself. I said, "No, thanks," and advised him that he too should quit. That incident has stayed with me. I would never return to smoking.

Nicotine Replacement Products

Most aids to quitting smoking are nicotine replacement products. They deliver small, steady doses of nicotine into the body to relieve some of the withdrawal symptoms, but without the buzz that keeps smokers hooked. Nicotine replacement products are now available in four forms: patches, gum, nasal spray, and inhalers. Like cigarettes, they deliver nicotine into the blood, but they don't contain the toxins and carcinogens that are largely responsible for cigarettes' dangerous health consequences.

Studies show nicotine replacement therapies may double the chances of success in quitting. Smokers should choose the method that appeals to them, and try another method if the first one doesn't work.

Nicotine patch: This transdermal system has been available since 1992 (over the counter since 1996). Each day, a new patch, which looks like a big bandage, is applied to a different area of dry, clean, nonhairy skin and left on for the amount of time recommended in the product's labeling. The patch may not be a good choice for those with skin problems or allergies to adhesive tape.

Nicotine gum: Approved by the FDA in 1996, the gum releases nicotine into the bloodstream through the lining of the mouth. You first chew it slowly until a slight tingling occurs, then it is placed between the cheek and teeth. Some gums contain about 2 mg of nicotine and can be used as a tapering-off measure. Studies indicate that a good percentage of the people who use this gum are helped. It is particularly valuable for people who quit smoking cold turkey. Chewing gum may not be a good choice for anyone with temporomandibular joint disease (TMJ), weak dental work, or dentures.

All of the nicotine replacements are powerful medications. Keep nicotine replacement products, including those that have been used and thrown away, out of reach of children and pets. Consult your doctor before making any choice that will affect your health.

The pill: The newest antismoking aid is a pill, Zyban (bupropion hydrochloride). It was approved by the FDA in 1997 and contains no nicotine. The active ingredient was originally approved as an antidepressant, but it does not work on people who are not clinically depressed. Some side effects from Zyban are dry mouth, sleeplessness, shakiness, and skin rash, and a small chance of a seizure.

Other methods: Hypnosis seminars and acupuncture are other methods that have been used to combat smoking. Other quitting systems, including support groups and counseling, are often available locally.

Behavior Modification Methods

In a study done about a decade ago using a program based on behavior modification and self-control techniques, 50 percent of the patients were smoke-free after a year. The degree of success was not gauged by the testimony of the smoker, but rather by blood studies. The blood of people who smoke contains a chemical—serum thiocyanate—that varies in proportion to the number of cigarettes smoked. Within fourteen days after quitting, most of the serum thiocyanate is gone from the blood. In the study's participants, the levels fell from a high to a normal range. Here are some behavior-training tips that may be useful.

Stimulus control: Remove yourself from situations that trigger the desire to light a cigarette. For example, if you always smoke when you sit down to watch TV, replace the cigarette with, say, a cup of tea.

Relaxation training: Instead of taking a cigarette, stand up and do some deep-breathing exercises. Think about something pleasant to allay anxiety. (See Chapter 25 for other ways to deal with stress.)

Thought stopping: If you find yourself saying, "I need a cigarette," replace that thought with something like, "If others can do without the weed, so can I."

Vitamins Help Quitters

A 1995 Scottish heart health study indicated that the combined dietary intakes of the antioxidant vitamins C and E and beta-carotene can change a smoker's behavior, as well as the health of both men and women subjects in the study.

Eating management: Avoid foods and food situations that trigger the desire to smoke. Don't sit down on your coffee break and pick up a cigarette. Change the pattern by eating an apple instead. Understand that you are deliberately doing this *instead* of smoking a cigarette.

Incompatible behavior: If you are eating candy or chewing on something, you cannot very easily smoke. Put on a binder clip—a small clip that goes on your lips—when you feel the urge to smoke.

Behavior rehearsal: Imagine nonsmoking behavior. Think of how nice it will be to kiss your loved one without worrying about smoker's breath. How liberating it will be to go places and sit in smoke-free planes, restaurants, or offices without obsessing on how to sneak a cigarette.

Cognitive coping: Think positively about quitting. See each day without cigarettes as a positive achievement in willpower and health. Feel good about yourself—quitting isn't easy.

Choose Your Time to Quit

When you are ready to quit smoking, pick a relatively nonstressful day. Unless you have an iron will, try not to quit during holiday seasons, when you are in the company of smokers and liable to be facing stress. Quitting during a stress-filled time or place might cause a smoking relapse.

Don't think of yourself as "denied" a pleasure. Your first goal should be to quit smoking and let your body heal from the effects of nicotine. When the tension gets too bad, get up and walk around your house, office, desk, or computer. Bend, breathe deeply, and distract yourself.

Cigarettes and Your Weight

Many people, especially young women, are concerned that they will gain weight if they stop smoking. This is a valid worry, since excess weight is a health concern too. However, you do not have to gain weight if you understand the problem. Most people who gain weight eat to overcome nicotine withdrawal symptoms or substitute food for cigarettes. There are ways to avoid or minimize weight gain.

Without nicotine in your body, you may experience short-term weight gain. Many physicians believe the weight you are when you quit is your normal weight. Water retention may also be noticed during the first week after quitting. This water retention, although usually only three to five pounds, is of concern for anyone with hypertension. Ask your doctor for suggestions to deal with this reaction when you quit.

Not everyone gains weight when they stop smoking. On average, though, smokers who quit gain about ten pounds. You are more likely to gain weight if you have smoked for ten to twenty years or smoked a pack or more each day. Although you might gain a few pounds, remember that you have stopped smoking for a healthier life.

Battling the Cravings

Once you stop smoking, it is important to learn how to handle cravings for cigarettes and food. A craving lasts only about five minutes, so you can probably distract yourself or wait it out. Here are some suggestions:

Replace smoking with other activities: Keep your hands busy. Doodle, work puzzles, knit, do needlepoint, or simply hold something. Greek worry beads might work.

Cut down on caffeine: Avoid beverages containing caffeine, and that includes many sodas. Nicotine withdrawal will make you feel jittery and nervous, and the caffeine will exacerbate those feelings.

Get enough rest: When you feel tired, you are more likely to crave cigarettes and food.

Reduce tension: To help relieve stress, relax by meditating, taking a walk, or even breathing deeply. Find something you enjoy thinking of; replace agitation with calm.

Get support and encouragement: Encourage friendship with people who do not smoke. You can also participate in smoke-free workshops.

Ask your doctor about nicotine replacement: If your withdrawal symptoms are severe, or you gain weight, get some professional help.

Don't tempt yourself: Keep a calendar or diary. Show the date you started to quit. If you do slip, ask yourself where you were, and what made you slip. Avoid similar situations in the future.

NOT EVEN ONE PUFF

Most people who abstain from smoking for three months can be cigarette-free for the rest of their lives. But after you've abstained for a while—even years—don't be lulled into taking a few puffs. The nature of nicotine addiction makes it hard to be an occasional smoker.

Other Smoking-Related Risks

SMOKE OF A DIFFERENT COLOR

A young woman was admitted to the hospital because of kidney stones. Although she was only twenty-two and quite thin, a medical exam showed her to have very high blood pressure. We could find no cause and eventually concluded that she had what is commonly called essential hypertension—high blood pressure due to no known cause.

In the course of treatment, the patient mentioned that she usually smoked marijuana daily. She had no access to the drug in the hospital, and her blood pressure gradually started to drop. She continued in my care for several months after her release from the hospital. Her blood pressure remained normal. The patient had stopped smoking anything.

As of now, there is no scientific evidence regarding the correlation between use of marijuana and high blood pressure, but this case struck me as pertinent and important. If you indulge, get your pressure checked by your doctor.

CAFFEINE CAUTIONS

The famous Native American hero Chief Crazy Horse was quoted as saying, "If the Great Spirit has something better than coffee, he keeps it for himself." Caffeine is in many beverages, and even in some over-the-counter

Fluttering Hearts

Here is a short list of caffeinated products:

BEVERAGES AND FOODS

Coffee (5 oz cup)	Regular, drip, 60–180 mg
	Regular, percolated, 40–170 mg
	Instant, regular, 30–120 mg
Tea (5 oz cup)	Brewed, 25–110 mg
Cola soft drinks (12 oz)	30–60 mg
Chocolate bar (average size)	30 mg

OVER-THE-COUNTER DRUGS (CHECK ALL LABELS)

No-Doz	200 mg
Excedrin	130 mg
Anacin, Empirin, Midol	65 mg

medicines such as painkillers, weight loss drugs, and cold remedies. Caffeine temporarily increases blood pressure. It is not thought harmful for people with normal blood pressure, but it may have a stronger and longer lasting effect on those with HBP, even at borderline levels. Moreover, coffee increases excretion of calcium, increasing the risk for high blood pressure. If you drink a caffeinated beverage, make sure you have an adequate calcium intake.

Essential to a healthy lifestyle is gaining control over negative or detrimental habits. Medical aids and behavioral techniques make quitting smoking easier than it was years ago. In addition to the dramatic improvement in their health, patients tell me they also have greater self-esteem and feel better about themselves since they stopped smoking.

CHAPTER 20

Alcohol and Illegal Drugs and Hypertension

The relationship between hypertension and excessive alcohol consumption has been recognized for almost a century. During this time, many scientific studies confirmed that alcoholism is a cause of hypertension, independent of any other factors, such as economic status, age, race, weight, serum cholesterol levels, or even tobacco use. If you drink excessively, your blood pressure will go up.

Effects of Alcohol on Your Body

One third of all American adults choose not to drink alcoholic beverages. Some people drink alcoholic beverages only once in a while. When you know the facts and effects of alcohol, you will be able to decide what is best for you. Alcohol is a drug. It affects the way you feel and affects every system in your body.

The most reasonable explanation for the hypertension associated with heavy drinking is alcohol's effect on the walls of the arteries. When alcohol is present in the bloodstream, it bathes the walls of the blood vessels, increasing their tension and thereby raising blood pressure. There are other complex explanations that support this hypothesis. According to one theory, alcohol blocks the passageway of chemicals into and out of the artery walls, tightening the walls and increasing blood pressure.

Moderation Is the Key

Until 1994, everyone seemed certain that any and all alcoholic beverages were detrimental. But then *The Journal of the American Medical Association* published an editorial with a surprising conjecture. If the entire population of the United States suddenly stopped drinking, there would be an additional 81,000 deaths due to heart disease each year. The article advised that abstaining from alcohol may be no better than drinking in moderation.

At the same time, Danish researchers were finishing a large study that followed the drinking habits of thirteen thousand people for more than a decade. To everyone's surprise, those who downed three to five glasses of wine daily had roughly half the risk of teetotalers of dying. The Harvard School of Public Health also weighed in: They said that the benefits of alcohol consumption (an enlargement of the blood vessels) disappear after as little as two drinks. It is generally thought that moderate drinking (usually defined as one or two drinks a day) helps prevent heart attacks and stroke.

FRENCH WINE

Although the French are known for serving rich pâté and buttery pastries, the French are not as likely to die from heart disease as other Westerners. The popularity of red wine among the French apparently explains the "French Paradox": a low rate of heart disease despite high-fat diets. Is wine better than beer or hard liquor? Wine drinkers appear to enjoy a slight edge: Wine grapes contain antioxidants that seem to prevent blood clots and arterial clogging, in combination with another chemical known to lower bad LDL cholesterol. One drink also raises blood levels of good HDL cholesterol. You'll get more antioxidants from red wine than white, because red is made from the whole grape. Another wine drinkers' bonus: Small amounts of alcohol may reduce the blood's tendency to form clots that can lead to heart attacks and strokes. Alcohol also slows the absorption of food, so if you drink a glass of wine with meals, you are less likely to send a sudden rush of sugar into the bloodstream, as usually occurs when you start eating.

Genes May Play a Part

Some experts suggest that there is a genetic predisposition to both hypertension and alcoholism. If so, how could one structure a study to determine the validity of this theory? One way might be to study a group of twins who had the same genetic background but who were raised separately. You would then need to have one twin who drinks and one who does not. On the surface, these sound like impossible conditions. However, just such a study was conducted in Sweden, where seventy pairs of identical male twins were studied. Each twin had been raised separately from the other. Blood pressure levels and alcohol consumption levels were compared for each set of twins, and the blood pressure reading was invariably higher in the twin who drank.

The results of this study indicate that the hypertension that accompanies alcoholism is an alcohol-induced rather than an inherited trait. Ultimately, however, for scientific purposes the number of people in this study is too small to be definitive, so the genetic factor cannot be ruled out. (When I first reviewed this study, I thought it was remarkable that the investigator had been able to find seventy pairs of twins who had been raised separately. Then it occurred to me that one of my own adopted children is one of a pair of twins who were separated at birth and raised apart.)

Effects on Long-term Drinkers

Various studies in England and Wales have demonstrated that long-term drinking invariably leads to hypertension and its various severe complications, such as stroke and heart attack. Another European study showed that the death rate from stroke was three times greater in heavy drinkers than in infrequent drinkers. In this study, high blood pressure was the cause of the strokes among the heavy drinkers.

In still other studies, the blood pressure levels of people who drank 60 ounces of hard liquor per month were twice that of those who drank less than 30 ounces of hard liquor a month.

Clinical Experiences

Even if all the scientific studies did not confirm that alcohol causes hypertension, you need only ask practicing physicians what their experience has

> ### Hypertension Risks
>
> From 5 to 11 percent of all hypertension in men is attributable to alcohol. The most common cause of irreversible hypertension in men is the consumption of more than 2 to 4 ounces of whiskey per day (or 8 to 16 ounces of wine, or 24 to 48 ounces of beer). A 1998 Harvard study found women who daily consume three or four beers or glasses of wine, or two mixed drinks, were 40 percent more likely to develop hypertension than low to moderate drinkers or abstainers. Drinking more would raise their risk even higher, to about 90 percent.

been. Most will acknowledge that when patients describe a pattern of heavy drinking, subsequent examination will reveal that they have high blood pressure.

Some of my patients tell me that they like to have a drink or two to help them relax; others drink because they find it hard to participate in social situations without a drink. Alcohol derives its relaxing effect by depressing the central nervous system. While one or two drinks may cause no harm in normal, healthy people, excessive or long-term use can lead to many problems. In social situations such as parties or working lunches, you should consider interspersing alcoholic drinks with soda or fruit juice.

Ability and special talent, however, are no protections against alcohol dependence. Geoff was a gifted writer and foreign correspondent when he became my patient. Geoff suffered from disastrously high blood pressure and was repeatedly warned about his drinking. Nonetheless, this talented writer would periodically go on binges. When he was sober, no amount of discussion could convince him of the self-destructiveness of his drinking. He continued to drink despite rising blood pressure levels until he was too sick to travel or work.

Drinking and Blood Pressure

ALCOHOL OVERLOADS THE LIVER

The body of the heavy drinker takes a severe beating. Most frequently damaged is the liver, because it is the organ responsible for getting alcohol out of the system. When excessive amounts of alcohol become concentrated in the liver, it causes real damage.

> ## Chronic Alcoholism and Other Diseases
>
> In the 1990s four European hypertension physicians joined together to study the relationship between alcohol and hypertension. They found that almost half of all heavy drinkers have arterial hypertension, which can be linked to heart rhythm problems and angina. The relationship between chronic alcohol consumption and HBP becomes obvious after age forty. Alcohol is the third associated risk factor for arterial hypertension after age and body weight, and ahead of tobacco and lifestyle. In other words, you can be thin, non-smoking, and a vegetarian, but your risk factor for hypertension will go up if you abuse alcohol.

About 80 percent of the cholesterol made by the liver is used to make bile. The liver also converts substances in digested food into proteins, fat, and carbohydrates. In heavy drinkers, the liver tries to burn off alcohol instead of processing fat, its usual job. As a result, the liver becomes infiltrated with fat. This leads first to hepatitis or inflammation of the liver, and finally to total liver damage. Since a properly functioning liver destroys many toxins in the body, when the liver itself is destroyed, many other systems become unbalanced.

ALCOHOL AND EPINEPHRINE AND SODIUM

But how does alcohol cause the blood pressure to rise? One theory is that the alcohol in your bloodsteam triggers the release of the hormone epinephrine (adrenaline), which narrows your blood vessels. We know that too much sodium produces an increase in blood pressure. Hypertension in beer drinkers may result from the large amount of sodium in beer. The sodium contained in six beers is sufficient to raise the blood pressure in those who are sodium-sensitive.

NUTRIENTS AND ALCOHOL

Eating a nutritious diet while reducing alcohol consumption can lower a heavy drinker's systolic pressure about 10 mm Hg and diastolic pressure about 7 mm Hg. One reason for this is that alcoholics don't generally get adequate nutrient levels of potassium, calcium, and magnesium.

HORMONE INTERACTION

Alcohol can damage the nerves that regulate the production of hormones. When this happens, the kidneys and adrenal glands, which produce the hormones that control blood pressure, are given no signal to stop, and therefore they overproduce. Hormonal overproduction may elevate blood pressure.

An October 1999 article in *The Journal of the American Medical Association* reports that postmenopausal women who drink alcohol while taking estrogen replacement therapy (ERT) may inadvertently raise the hormone level in their blood. Though estrogen makes the arteries more flexible, increased estrogen levels have been linked to high blood pressure. Some experts believe that in this way estrogen encourages the body to retain liquid; that additional liquid may put additional stress on arteries and raise the risk of hypertension.

YOUR BRAIN ON ALCOHOL

The interaction between the psychological and emotional factors in drinking and hypertension is not completely understood. It is possible that the relationship is reversed: Hypertension occurs first and excessive drinking follows. The drinking can be a need for relief from internal pressure. Certain driven and success-oriented people might develop hypertension and then turn to drinking to relax.

The chances of a cerebrovascular accident in the twenty-four hours following a heavy drinking episode can reach 33 percent, according to a 1996 study in Sweden and the United States. The study also indicates cerebral hemorrhage and cerebral infarction (stroke) accidents are more frequent in alcoholics than in nondrinkers. The main cause of this is arterial hypertension, cardiac rhythm problems, and the direct effect of alcohol on cerebral vessels.

How Much Is Too Much?

Just how much alcohol does a person have to consume daily to be called a heavy drinker? Anything in excess of moderate drinking must be considered heavy drinking. Moderation is no more than one drink per day for women and no more than two drinks per day for men. Count as a drink:

12 ounces of regular beer (150 calories)

5 ounces of wine (100 calories)

1.5 ounces of 80-proof distilled spirits (100 calories)

Medications, Alcohol, and High Blood Pressure

Alcohol also can cause personality changes and can destroy the proper functioning of the nervous system. How does this happen? Normally the brain cells, or neurons, communicate with one another through electrical

---

A Drinker's Questionnaire

How can you tell if you are an alcoholic? Finding a simple answer might seem difficult, but Dr. John A. Ewing of the University of North Carolina at Chapel Hill has provided an excellent yardstick. Answer the following four questions:

1. Have you ever felt you ought to cut down on your drinking?

2. Have people annoyed you by criticizing your drinking?

3. Have you ever felt bad or guilty about your drinking?

4. Have you ever had a drink first thing in the morning—an eye-opener to steady your nerves?

If you answer yes to any two of these questions, you should stop drinking and seek help. Your doctor will be able to help you. Here are some other resources:

◆ Alcoholics Anonymous (AA): a voluntary fellowship of alcoholics who help themselves and each other get and stay sober. Check your local phone book for a chapter, or call 212-870-3400.

◆ The National Institute on Alcohol Abuse and Alcoholism (NIAAA): 301-443-3860.

◆ The National Council on Alcoholism and Drug Dependence can refer you to treatment centers: 800-622-2255.

Alcohol Interactions with Over-the-Counter Pain Relievers

OTCS	CAN CAUSE
*NSAIDs: Advil, Aleve.	Stomach and intestinal bleeding to varying degrees
Non-NSAIDs: Tylenol	Chronic alcohol abuse has been associated with liver complications
Antihistamines: Benadryl	Sedative effect, drowsiness, confusion

*NSAIDs are nonsteroidal anti-inflammatory drugs, such as aspirin.

Note: If you have any questions about interactions between alcohol and medicines, your doctor is your best source of advice.

impulses or the passage of various chemical molecules that act as messengers. These impulses and molecules pass from cell to cell, moving within the liquid medium of each cell. When alcohol is in this liquid, it produces physical changes. The viscosity or thickness of the fluid is altered so that the passage of electrical impulses and molecules is delayed, slowed, or even prevented. This obstruction accounts for the depression of brain activity. When drinking continues over time, the changes that occur in the liquid medium are more permanent. It is possible that long-term damage to the nervous system is a reason for the development of hypertension.

One of the most insidious aspects of alcohol consumption is that alcohol is often included in common over-the-counter medications and other products.

Illegal Drugs and High Blood Pressure

As we have seen, alcohol and many prescription drugs, as well as over-the-counter drugs, can affect your blood pressure. The right medications can make you feel better, function better, and contribute to your health. The wrong drugs, however, especially illegal ones, can send your blood pressure soaring.

Illegal drugs can vary in potency and can be toxic to many of the body's vital systems. Here is an overview of some of the disastrous health effects of some illegal drugs:

Marijuana: Even in small doses marijuana can impair memory function. Health effects also include accelerated heartbeat and increased blood pressure.

Cocaine: A very strong stimulant to the nervous system, including the brain, this drug produces an accelerated heart rate at the same time as it constricts the blood vessels; this causes the temperature and blood pressure to rise.

Heroin: An illegal opiate that causes shallow breathing, nausea, panic, insomnia, and the need for increasingly higher doses. Withdrawal symptoms include tremors, panic, chills, sweating, nausea, and elevations in blood pressure, pulse, and respiratory rate.

Methamphetamine: This is a powerful stimulant. Amphetamine cousins are sometimes included in "under-the-counter" diet pills and should be avoided. Side effects of methamphetamine include hot flashes, dryness of the mouth, sweating, palpitations, and hypertension.

While alcohol in moderate amounts may not be harmful for most people, for those with hypertension overuse of alcohol could be deadly. Use common sense and the advice of your physician to help you limit, if not eliminate, alcohol from your lifestyle.

CHAPTER 21

Sleeping with Hypertension

Sleep apnea is a common problem that causes breathing to stop during sleep. The sleeper never wakes, but doesn't breathe for periods of up to two minutes, many times during a night. Sleep apnea occurs when the respiratory muscles do not function as they should, and obstructive sleep apnea happens when the flow of air through the neck passage is blocked. An August 2000 study at Penn State College of Medicine indicates that hypertension risks increase with the severity of sleep problems.

There is a relationship between heavy body weight, sleep apnea, and high blood pressure. They are linked in a complicated relationship, and sleep apnea is often ignored. One of the more common patterns: First a person gains weight, then the weight gain brings on sleep apnea (usually obstructive apnea).

Obstructive Sleep Apnea

This is the most common and most severe form of sleep apnea. It is also called upper-airway apnea. The soft palate, located at the base of the tongue, and the uvula (the little dab of fleshy tissue that hangs from the center of the soft palate) relax and sag, obstructing the airway and making breathing labored and noisy. Snoring can result. When breathing stops periodically, a listener hears the snoring broken by pauses. A collapse of the airway walls blocks breathing entirely. As pressure to breathe builds, blood pressure builds.

More than 20 million Americans suffer from sleep apnea, yet only 5 per-

> ### Breathe Deeply
>
> If you suffer from high blood pressure and insomnia, the reason could be that you periodically stop breathing during sleep. A 1999 report from researchers at the Laboratory for the Diagnosis of Sleep Disorders in Israel noted that just a moment or two without a breath can nudge your blood pressure into the stratosphere.

cent have been diagnosed and are being treated, according to the National Sleep Disorders Research Center. Your answers to this short sleep quiz will help you decide whether you or someone close to you suffers from sleep apnea, which may affect blood pressure.

1. Are you a loud habitual snorer, disturbing your bedroom companion?
2. Do you feel tired and groggy on awakening?
3. Do you experience sleepiness and fatigue during waking hours?
4. Are you overweight?
5. Have you been observed to choke, gasp, or hold your breath during sleep?

If your answer to any of the above is yes, you should discuss your symptoms with your physician, or write the American Sleep Apnea Association, P.O. Box 66, Belmont, MA 02178.

Dr. Anthony Kales in Hershey, Pennsylvania, examined fifty middle-aged people chosen because their sleep blood pressure was in the hypertensive range. Each of these men's and women's sleep was monitored in the sleep laboratory. It turned out that about one in three had sleep apnea. The good news is that there are many cases in which hypertension is secondary to sleep apnea. When the sleep apnea is treated, the blood pressure decreases to normal levels.

A Good Night's Sleep

Most people with sleep apnea benefit from the following suggestions.

◆ Weight loss may help in the treatment of sleep apnea, while lowering blood pressure. Even a partial weight loss (20 pounds by a 200-pound

> ### Research Never Sleeps
>
> For a sleep study, Swedish scientists developed what they called a respiratory disturbance index. They asked the subjects about symptoms that could indicate a sleep disorder, such as snoring, breathing stoppages, sleepiness, and falling asleep while driving. Researchers also looked at cholesterol levels, blood gas readings, blood pressure, and resting heart rate. The more than a thousand subjects were given devices to monitor their breathing. After analyzing the results, the researchers concluded that those with a high disturbance index had high blood pressure and heart rates. Experts said that patients with high blood pressure who showed symptoms of sleep disorder should tell their doctors—immediately.

man, who should weigh about 170, for instance) may improve breathing during sleep and make sleep more restful.

- Drinking alcoholic beverages within two hours of bedtime should be avoided. Alcohol depresses breathing and makes apnea more frequent and severe. According to the American Sleep Disorders Association, alcohol can trigger an apnea in people who would otherwise merely snore.

- Don't take any sleeping pills, even mild or over-the-counter pills, unless you have discussed your sleep patterns and how they might relate to your HBP with your doctor. Discuss any other medications you may be taking at the same time. Interestingly, medications to relieve congestion of the nose may be helpful in reducing the likelihood of apnea. A new adhesive strip that is worn across the nose during sleep to keep the nostrils open may work.

- Exercise during the day, and try to get outside in daylight. It will keep your sleep pattern normal. Keep a regular schedule.

- Avoid caffeine within several hours of bedtime.

- Don't smoke cigarettes to help you sleep. Nicotine is a stimulant. And smoking is dangerous; the hazard of falling asleep with a burning cigarette is very real.

- Sleep position plays a part. Back sleepers have a higher incidence of

> ## A Sleep Herb
>
> Lavender, which was used to perfume baths and underwear of the Romans, has been used for over a thousand years in various folk remedies. It has been studied for its sedative effect at the University of Leicester in England. Researchers introduced lavender-scented oils into the living quarters of elderly people. The lavender oil seems to have a light sedative effect and encourages sleep.

apnea than side sleepers. Pillows placed behind the back or a tennis ball attached to the back of your pajamas will encourage side sleeping.

- Most of all, follow your antihypertension program.

If you are tired during the day and cannot function normally because you don't sleep restfully, and if this fatigue lasts for more than two or three weeks, you should see your doctor. For general information about sleep, contact the Better Sleep Council, P.O. Box 13, Washington, DC 20044.

CHAPTER 22

Hypertension and Aging

Since 1900 the percentage of Americans older than 65 years has tripled, and the number has increased tenfold, to about 32 million people. The older population itself is also living longer. The U.S. Census Bureau estimates that more than 16 million Americans will be older than 85 by the year 2050. High blood pressure can affect people of all ages, but most people with the problem seem to be over the age of 40; two thirds of those between ages 65 and 74, and three quarters of those more than 75, have elevated blood pressure. High blood pressure, however, should not be viewed as a normal and inevitable part of aging.

Treatment Benefits

Treatment of hypertension in older people has demonstrated major benefits. Large trials of patients older than age 60 have shown that antihypertension therapy (nondrug and, when needed, drug therapy) reduces the incidence of stroke, cardiovascular disease, and heart failure.

Primary (essential) hypertension is by far the most common form of hypertension in older people. Physicians recognize that other identifiable causes of hypertension may occur more frequently in older people. The causes may include, among other factors, atherosclerosis and hypertension brought on by kidney problems. These additional or triggering causes are most often seen in people whose hypertension is first diagnosed after age 60, or if the hypertension is resistant to treatment.

Watch Your Systolic Pressure

Since it is obvious that there is a prevalence of hypertension in the elderly in the United States, some generalizations may be made about the health risks of elderly hypertensive persons: They have a risk for cardiovascular death, and a death rate twice that of elderly persons with normal blood pressure. The risk of stroke is also three times greater than for those with normal blood pressure. Elderly people with high systolic hypertension and normal diastolic pressure are at just as great, or greater, risk for cardiovascular events and stroke than those with normal pressure. Systolic blood pressure may be the most important risk factor.

Mature Management

Older people, because they visit their doctors more frequently, are more likely than young people to be aware they have HBP. They are also more likely to adhere to therapy and to achieve better control of their blood pressure than our younger patients. Nonetheless, I am always aware of certain physical, medical, psychological, and social factors among my elderly patients that can affect adherence to the treatment of other problems they may have.

Physical and Medical Factors

A number of physical or medical factors can impact hypertension treatment and control among elderly patients. If you are elderly, you and your caregiver (if you have one) should consider these points:

- You are more likely than younger hypertensives to take multiple prescriptions and over-the-counter medications; this causes a risk of harmful drug interactions.

- Problems with hearing or eyesight can make instructions difficult for some to understand and carry out. Repeat your understanding of the directions to your doctor or pharmacist so these health care providers can clarify any points that seem difficult.

- Your diet may be deficient in fresh fruits and vegetables (about 75 percent of all adult Americans should eat more fresh fruits and vegetables).

Taking the Blood Pressure of the Elderly

According to a 1997 report from the National Institutes of Health, blood pressure must be measured in older persons with special care because some older people may have falsely high sphygmomanometer readings. This is thought to be due to excessive vascular stiffness. In addition, more older people with hypertension, especially women, seem to have white coat hypertension.

Nutritional guides are throughout this book, and you can contact the National Institute on Aging Information Center at 800-222-2225. Check the DASH diet in Chapter 10 and Appendix 2, and some of the recipes in Chapter 33. If you have special nutrition needs, or are limited in your ability to grocery-shop or prepare and consume food, check the food services for the elderly in your local area.

- Even mild cognitive dysfunction or depression, or a memory lapse, must be considerations in deciding the appropriate antihypertensive therapy for you. You must be able to carry out a long-term treatment that is practical, safe, and effective.

- If you have difficulty in opening safety caps, it may hinder adherence to a hypertension program that includes medications; you should report such problems to your physician or caregiver.

Evaluating an elderly patient's ability to understand and participate in treatment is time well spent. Evidence now shows that treatment can be initiated and maintained without an increase in dementia or depression and without much negative effect on abilities.

Happiness Is Important

We're all getting older. A number of psychological and social factors may impede the adherence to therapy among older people. Here are some points you or someone you care about should consider:

- In many older married couples, the wife is the medical caregiver. It has been my nonscientific observation that many men, particularly widowers, don't take control of their own health as they should.

- Many elderly people live alone. Having little contact with family or friends to ask about health and treatment can hinder adherence to therapy. Building a support system is as important in later years as it was in other times of life. It requires an effort, but it's well worth it. If you do live alone, get to know a neighbor; most people are flattered and happy to be asked for help. Participating in holiday celebrations and traditional days with a group will enhance your enjoyment of life.

- A low fixed income and the limitations of health insurance benefits can discourage elderly patients from acquiring prescribed medications, keeping appointments, or obtaining routine or special laboratory tests. The paperwork for insurance payments or Medicare and Medicaid payments can be frustrating; call your local Social Security office or contact the National Institute on Aging Information Center, P.O. Box 8057, Gaithersburg, MD 20898; 800-222-2225, TTY: 800-222-4225.

- Transportation problems, particularly during the colder months and often coupled with fear of crime, keep many older patients away from sources of medical help.

- Flexibility in scheduling visits and marking a special calendar will help you achieve better control over your life. I find that a little extra time and attention to the elderly living alone often increases that patient's adherence to treatment. In a number of my patients, follow-up visits needed to stabilize blood pressure have had to be balanced against their financial limitations and transportation problems. You, or your caregiver, should take advantage of home care services, community blood pressure programs, local health departments, or public health nursing facilities.

Life Quality Counts

Very little information about the effect of hypertensive medications on the quality of life of older patients is available. A recent study has reported no evidence of negative effects on physical, social, intellectual, or emotional functions, but it points out that no information about life quality specific to the elderly has yet been published.

From my own many years of experience as a physician, I can tell you that nondrug methods to control high blood pressure can be successful for every age group. All have positive outcomes for health and well-being in just about everyone.

One of the most depressing aspects of aging is the feeling of loss of control that affects people who feel their vigor and power waning. Taking control of your life through your own efforts, and seeing your efforts rewarded, will improve your quality of life.

CHAPTER 23

Women and High Blood Pressure

While both men and women develop high blood pressure, I have noticed no significant gender difference in responses and outcomes. However, there are a few areas in gender that do make a difference. Primarily, women should be particularly on guard against the early onset of hypertension. Three of every four women with high blood pressure know they have it. Yet studies indicate that fewer than one in three women are controlling their hypertension.

An Equal Opportunity Disease

Although most women think that the leading cause of death among women is cancer, it's actually heart disease, which affects 35 percent of all women. One in ten American women 45 to 64 years of age has some form of heart disease, and this increases to one in four in women over 65. Another two million women have had a stroke. Both heart disease and stroke are serious disorders involving the blood vessels.

Just as with men, high blood pressure greatly increases the chance of developing heart disease and is the most important risk factor for stroke for women. Even slightly elevated levels can double a woman's risk and also increase the chance of developing congestive heart failure and kidney disease. More than half of American women—and 70 percent of African-American women—will develop high blood pressure at some time in their lives.

What Can a Woman Do?

If you have high blood pressure, you can control it with proper treatment. You can help to prevent and control high blood pressure by taking the following basic blood-pressure-lowering steps:

- Limit your alcohol use.
- Use less salt and sodium.
- Be physically active.
- Lose weight, but take it slowly.
- Eat for health.
- Quit smoking.
- Iron: For women, the recommended daily allowance for iron is 15 milligrams per day. Young women lose iron each month during menstruation. After menopause, body iron stores generally begin to increase.
- Note: Keep milk on the menu. Don't cut out dairy products in trying to reduce calories and fat. Dairy products are rich in calcium and are important for women. Instead choose nonfat or low-fat dairy products. In addition to dairy foods, other sources of calcium include salmon, tofu, broccoli, and calcium-enriched orange juice and food products.

Hypertension and Oral Contraceptives

Women taking oral contraceptives experience a small but detectable increase in both systolic and diastolic pressure. Hypertension is two or three times more common in women taking oral contraceptives, especially obese women and those over 35. Women age 35 and older who smoke cigarettes and take oral contraceptives should make extra efforts to quit smoking.

If hypertension develops when you take oral contraceptives, talk with your physician about stopping the hormone replacements. Blood pressure will normalize in most cases. If high blood pressure persists, or if pregnancy poses greater risks for hypertension, you and your doctor might find other more acceptable contraceptive methods. A prudent watch-and-see approach when an oral contraceptive is used is a good idea. Some physicians prescribe no more than a six-month supply at any time, and measure a patient's blood pressure on a semiannual basis.

Hypertension and Hormones

Hypertension has many causes, and some physicians think that women's natural estrogen dominance is one of them. They believe the estrogen dominance and oral contraceptive agents may lead to water retention, which can lead to high blood pressure. Since the extra water is contained within body cells and not in extracellular spaces, it is not effectively reduced by diuretics. In women not on contraceptive pills, estrogen dominance may sometimes be synonymous with progesterone deficiency. When progesterone is supplied, weight goes down (excess water is excreted) and blood pressure returns to normal.

High Blood Pressure Linked with Bone Loss in Women

According to a 1999 article in *Science News*, researchers discovered that women with a systolic blood pressure reading of 148 or more had an average bone density loss equal to 0.6 percent of their bone mass each year. In contrast, women with a systolic reading of less than 124 suffered bone loss at about half that rate. Good news: 15 percent of women in the study on hormone replacement therapy had about half as much bone loss, on average, as those who did not take estrogen replacement. Further research indicates a relationship between salt intake and calcium loss. Salt gradually siphons calcium out of the body, and high-salt diets often accompany bone loss.

CHAPTER 24

Impotence and Hypertension

Impotence is not a disease, but a condition brought on by one or more health problems. It is a side effect, a symptom of other problems. Thirty years ago, when men went to their doctors asking for help with erectile problems, they were told that there was no treatment, because the problem was caused by aging or nerves, or some kind of repressed emotions.

As doctors learned more through research, they developed a pharmaceutical solution for many men. A visit to your doctor can often solve or ameliorate the problem.

Until recently, few people—even physicians—spoke publicly about impotence, but it never has been rare. An estimated 20 to 30 million men in the United States suffer impotence; this translates to one in five men, or about 16 percent of the entire U.S. population. Note: A study found that women with high blood pressure, regardless of whether they took medication, found it difficult to achieve sexual satisfaction and had impaired vaginal lubrication. It seems lowering blood pressure is good for the gander, and is also good for the goose.

HBP and ED (Erectile Dysfunction)

Physicians and medical researchers who have studied the physiological and psychological responses involved in male sexuality divide impotence into three areas for treatment:

> ## *Licorice Is Not a Love Candy*
>
> If you eat large quantities of licorice every day, you may run a risk of developing high blood pressure and heart disease. Licorice or licorice extract causes your body to retain sodium and fluids and to lose potassium, which raises blood pressure and puts a strain on the heart. In a letter in *The New England Journal of Medicine*, three Italian physicians reported that licorice root may also impede sexual performance and even cause a loss of sex drive in men. The doctors found that the testosterone levels of a group of men in a study decreased during the period they ate licorice. The doctors concluded: "Men with decreased libido or other sexual dysfunction, as well as those with hypertension, should be aware of licorice side effects."

Physical causes, which account for about 85 to 90 percent of the
   problems

Psychological causes, which account for about 10 percent

Problems of undetermined origin, which account for about
   5 percent

A number of physical causes, many linked with illnesses such as diabetes, heart and vascular disease, hypertension and antihypertensive medications, prostate cancer, pelvic trauma and surgery, are implicated. Many medications used to treat hypertension will actually cause sexual impotence. It is medical knowledge that over two hundred known prescribed medications can trigger impotence, including some antihypertensive medications.

Usually, physical impotence develops over a period of time. It can involve any or all of these problems:

* Inability to initiate an erection that results from impaired release of the chemicals sent to the penis. The problem can develop from insufficient hormones, spinal cord injury, radical pelvic surgery, or neurological disease.

* Poor blood flow into the penis. The inability to develop an erection can be caused by blockage in the arteries, hypertension, smoking, diabetes,

and vascular problems brought on by high cholesterol as well as pelvic trauma.

♦ Blood that escapes too quickly from the penis, leaking back into the vascular system. This inability to maintain an erection is common in cases of hypertension, smoking, diabetes, high cholesterol, and pelvic trauma as well as other causes.

Most medical scientists believe that about 33 percent of these problems come from diseases of the blood vessels (hypertension among them), and about 25 percent from diabetes mellitus. It is wise to remember that some physical causes of impotence are beyond your control. Diabetes, high blood pressure, stroke, or prostate disease are difficult to treat, and difficult to live with. Feeling responsible for their symptoms is not appropriate.

Physiological Causes

Hypertension, a disease of the vascular system, can interfere with the passage of blood. Since erection depends on a flow of blood into the penis, hypertension can cause sexual impotency.

Think about it this way: If poor blood flow occurs in the heart or coronary vessels, it causes heart attacks; when it occurs in the brain, it causes strokes; when it occurs in the penis, it causes impotence.

Diabetes is a very common cause of impotence. This disease can damage both blood vessels and nerves. When the nerves are affected, the brain cannot properly transmit a sexual stimulus. The neurological diseases that can cause impotence are multiple sclerosis, Parkinson's disease, and spinal cord

---

A Neighbor's Problems

For many years my office was in a residential building. I got to know many other tenants, and a neighbor came to see me for a minor complaint. As always, I checked his blood pressure and noted that it was through the roof. He explained that his business had gone into bankruptcy and he was also having sexual problems. We worked together and gradually lowered his blood pressure; with lowered BP, his sexual problem abated. He reported that Viagra did not help his impotency—but lowering blood pressure did. Note: Viagra will not overcome impotence due to hypertension.

injury. Deficiencies in the endocrine system that cause low levels of testosterone (the male sexual hormone) and of a thyroid hormone often cause poor-quality erections. Radical pelvic surgery may result in impotence. Surgery involving the prostate gland, the bladder, or colon may sever the nerves involved in erection.

Age may be a factor. According to the 1,200-man Massachusetts Male Aging Study in 1989, the amount of blood in a man's penis, all-important for a firm erection, declines decade by decade. So too does the uptilt angle of his erection, the amount and force of ejaculate, and the length of the orgasm. The changes are mainly due to vascular problems. A greater thickening and hardening of the arterial walls (atherosclerosis) has been measured in the penis than in any other parts of the body.

Self-Inflicted Problems

You can also do it to yourself: Overuse of prescription drugs and substance abuse—from illegal drugs to the excessive use of alcohol and cigarettes—are enemies of an active sex life. Nicotine narrows the blood vessels that provide blood to the penis, and excessive alcohol use can damage the blood vessels and nerves involved in achieving an erection.

Treatments and Claims

Since sexuality is a vital part of life, 36,000 prescriptions for Viagra were written in the first two weeks after it received government approval. It has continued at the rate of about 10,000 pills a day. However, the pills are expensive (about $12 each), and certainly not for everyone. In the spring of 1998, over 130 Americans who took this popular impotence drug died. The majority of the deaths were from heart attacks—highlighting the need for careful use of *any* medication.

Since these tragedies, Pfizer, the manufacturer of Viagra, has instituted a new warning label, and the Food and Drug Administration has alerted doctors to be cautious about prescribing Viagra, especially for men who recently have had heart attacks or who have very high blood pressure.

The new Viagra guidelines say that the drug is not safe for use by heart patients who take organic nitrates, including nitroglycerin patches or tablets. They also recommend a complete medical checkup prior to drug use for those who have had chest pain or other signs of poor blood flow to the heart; who have congestive heart failure and low blood pressure; or who are taking drugs to control high blood pressure, kidney or liver disease, or multiple sclerosis. According to Victor Contreras, M.D., writing in *The Journal of Longevity,* negative reactions can also include vision disturbances, headaches, and priapism (a condition involving abnormal and painful erections). Viagra, in combination with antihypertensive medications or nitroglycerin, may cause fainting.

BUYER BEWARE

Unfortunately, false hope sometimes sells. Fraud is packaged in exotic pills or in miracle cures. It encourages wishful thinking and thrives on desperation and fear. Impotence is a medical condition for which treatments are available from qualified health care practitioners. Don't be embarrassed to talk to your doctor—you are not alone. The Federal Trade Commission offers these tips for evaluating all medical claims; here are some of the ploys you should be aware of:

- If a product is advertised as "effective" but no physician's prescription is necessary, forget it.
- If the product is a "breakthrough" that no one else seems to know about, check with your doctor.
- If the product is promoted by a medical organization you have never heard of, check with your doctor.
- Such claims as "scientifically proven" and "proven in clinical studies" should make you suspicious.
- Terms such as "natural" and "herbal" do not mean that the product is effective or harmless, or without side effects that you may not want.

CHAPTER 25

Stress and Hypertension

S tress is a part of life. Daily events—stress—challenge mental, physical, and emotional stability. Stress falls into some general categories. There are the life stresses, because just living brings many changes and challenges. Life stresses can include everything from a happy holiday to the death of a beloved friend. A stress scale of these life stresses was developed by psychologists in 1967. Health problems, social problems, new employment, changes in living conditions are all very stressful. The death of a spouse is thought to be the highest stress, but even Christmas is listed on this stress scale.

Some stresses come from within. Excessive demands that you may make on yourself, or demands from others, add to your level of stress. Stress affects every part of your body, and your blood pressure is particularly vulnerable.

Hans Selye, the Stress Definer

In the early 1930s, Hans Selye, M.D., a medical researcher, noted what he called the stress syndrome. We also call this the fight-or-flight reaction. When faced with stress, your body gears up to face the danger or insult, the fight response, or it gathers strength to run away, the flight response.

The stress hormone adrenaline, along with several other hormones, travels through your body to increase your blood pressure and heart rate, speed your breathing rate, increase blood sugar, and alter other body processes. For example, the fat cells release fats into the bloodstream to increase available energy for use by your muscles. All this prepares you to meet danger: Your body is alert, aroused, and tense. Once the encounter is over, your body relaxes and hormone levels and other systems return to normal.

When stress becomes particularly onerous or prolonged, the fight-or-flight response can become harmful. Stress and how you react to it can determine whether it will lead to high blood pressure. How you deal with stress is often learned behavior; if you are not dealing with stress in a way that relieves it, then you can learn new ways. Becoming adept at handling the stress in your life may lower your blood pressure.

Adaptation Leads to Hypertension

How does stress translate into hypertension? Hans Selye's fight-or-flight reaction may be the answer. When the body is experiencing stress it makes internal changes. One way is to increase the blood pressure within the arterial system to increase the supply of nutrients and oxygen to the muscles and the brain. When confronted by stress, the body responds with a rise in blood pressure.

Eventually, if this is repeated often enough, the arteries attempt to protect themselves from the increased pressure on their walls and go into a spasm—a tightening of the artery walls similar to tightening your fist. This narrowing brings about a further increase in pressure, causing more spasms. Let's use our image of a garden hose once more to help us understand this response. Imagine you are holding a soft hose in your hand. Tighten your fist around the hose: You are now producing a situation similar to spasms in the artery. A vicious cycle develops: more pressure, more spasms, causing increased pressure.

The vascular system is a series of pipes and tubes with areas that act as valves, causing an increase in resistance and thereby an increase in pressure. If you rest, you decrease the need for blood to pass through the system. Thus you decrease the demand for pressure. The more relaxation, the less need for blood flow, and the greater the drop in pressure. It has been commonly observed that in hospital patients short periods of bed rest will reduce blood pressure levels. True, the reduction is not very pronounced in older patients or in patients who have prolonged and severely elevated blood pressure, but it does hold true for the younger patients whose blood

> ## Mark's Case
>
> Mark, a student in a local university, studied late into the night and devoted his weekends to doing research. He never socialized or took a vacation: there was so much work to be done and there was so little time.
>
> After college, Mark went to medical school. However, he felt ill equipped to deal with many of life's frustrating and complex problems, and secretly he feared he was not sufficiently skilled. Uncomfortable dealing with people, Mark joined a pharmaceutical company as a researcher. His workday extended from early morning until midnight and his efforts resulted in many of the company's new drugs. After a promotion, however, Mark suddenly experienced chest pains but refused to acknowledge them and worked even harder. As Mark's blood pressure inched upward, he was stricken with a fatal heart attack, a tragic ending to a high-pressured life.

pressure still can be corrected. Simple physical rest is important. The greater the degree of rest, the better the response.

Stress and Personality Types

Mark, a type A personality, was highly motivated, internally stressed, constantly striving toward greater and greater accomplishments. Mark's way is the type A way of dealing with stress. At the other end of the behavior spectrum is the type B personality, an easygoing, low-key individual, contemplative, relaxed, and often passive. Unlike the type A personality, the type B personality is not usually internally stressed.

It would be convenient if we could divide people into type A and type B personalities, but it isn't that easy. There are many type A individuals with normal blood pressure, just as there are seemingly relaxed people with high blood pressure.

TYPE A AND TYPE B

The idea of just two personality types—type A and type B—is an oversimplification, and may not be a correct understanding of personality and its relationship to stress. Most people are not pure A or pure B but rather a

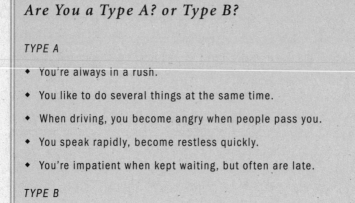

Are You a Type A? or Type B?

TYPE A

- You're always in a rush.
- You like to do several things at the same time.
- When driving, you become angry when people pass you.
- You speak rapidly, become restless quickly.
- You're impatient when kept waiting, but often are late.

TYPE B

- You like games where everyone wins.
- You're fairly content in your life.
- You take your time when eating, and enjoy dinner out.
- You love jokes and enjoy laughter.
- If you miss a deadline, you're not overly upset.

blend of both, with a greater propensity toward one or the other. Not all doctors agree on the importance of these two descriptive types, but there is enough evidence that they may be useful.

TRAITS OR LIFESTYLE? OR BOTH?

Anyone who has raised more than one child knows that each child has a unique personality. Even as toddlers, some are very serious about almost everything, while others don't seem to worry. Although it is possible to modify our personality traits, most personalities seem to remain essentially unchanged during our lifetime.

Some people seem to be born with a tendency to be stressed, no matter what situations they encounter. The individual response to pressure is determined by the relationship between the amount of stress that is present from an external force or activity and the internal stress response that exists within each person. The effect of stress on blood pressure can be seen in light of three factors: genetic predisposition, lifestyle habits, and allowing the high blood pressure to continue.

- Individual stress involves a genetically programmed personality. ("You're just like your grandmother.") Has anyone said something like that to you when you were a child? Maybe you are just like some relative.

- Stress is also affected by a stimulus to raise your blood pressure. (No one in your family has high blood pressure, but you are overweight; you salt every food and seldom walk anyplace, much less get any exercise.)

- Even though you have high blood pressure, you don't take anything to control it or lower it, allowing it to zoom out of control (A buffet table full of cheeses, sausage, and pickles is hard to resist.)

STRESS IS UNIVERSAL

Stress is with us all the time, but what stresses us varies from person to person. What may relax one person may be stressful to another. If you are an active person who likes to keep busy all the time, taking it easy at the beach on a beautiful day may feel extremely frustrating, nonproductive, upsetting—and stressful.

Here's an example of this from my own experience. When Diana, a thirty-four-year-old stockbroker, came for a routine medical exam, she had high blood pressure. When I couldn't find any medical cause, I considered her background and daily routine. Diana's job required that she make far-reaching decisions that involved large sums of money. Any error in judgment could result in substantial losses, a failure that would be noted immediately. It seemed to me that her stressful job clearly was the cause of the high blood pressure. Yet I was forced to question my own explanation a month later.

Stress and the Executive Myth

We usually think that heads of large corporations, surgeons who hold life in their hands, and race car drivers work in stressful situations. However, recent research lists being a waitress as among the most stressful of occupations. Caught between the cook and the customer, a waitress is under stress from both. Furthermore, low wages, low status, and little respect from customers are part of the equation. The biggest problem is that a waitress has very few ways of controlling her stress.

Diana referred her co-worker William to me. This young man's blood pressure was well below what is considered normal, yet he had the same job as Diana, with the same responsibilities. Their work was identical. If external stress alone were the causative agent in hypertension, William should also have had high blood pressure. Yet he did not.

Diana and William were about the same age, but that's where the similarity ended. Unlike Diana, William came from an easygoing family and he remembered his father observing that "life is too short to be upset." Diana was nervous and tense, whereas William was very relaxed. On that basis alone, one could have chosen which person had hypertension. The stress associated with the job was only a secondary factor. The primary factor was the difference in temperament and how each person dealt with stress. These two cases suggest that external stress alone does not cause hypertension.

Reacting and Adapting to Stress

To use stress in a positive way and prevent it from becoming distress, or "bad stress," you should become aware of your own reactions to stressful events. The body responds to stress by going through three states: alarm, resistance, exhaustion. For example, let's consider what happens to a commuter in rush-hour traffic. If a car suddenly cuts in front of our commuter, his initial alarm reaction may include fear of an accident, anger at the other driver, and general frustration. The commuter's body responds with an alarm stage by releasing hormones into the bloodstream. The next stage is resistance, in which the body repairs damage caused by stress. If the stress of rush-hour commuter driving continues with repeated close calls or traffic jams, his body will not have time to make repairs. The commuter may then become conditioned to expect problems when driving. The commuter will feel stressed at the beginning of each commute, even if there is no reason. Eventually, our commuter may develop a physical problem that is related to stress such as migraine headaches, high blood pressure, backaches, or insomnia. While it is impossible to live free of stress and distress, it is possible to prevent some distress and to minimize its impact when the stress can't be avoided.

SHORT-TERM AND LONG-TERM STRESS

Some years ago, during the Korean War, I served as a medical officer on the battleship *Wisconsin*. We were subject to all the stress that actual battle conditions produce. My battle station was in the ship's sick bay, a number of decks below the waterline.

During action, this area was sealed off so that if the ship was hit by a torpedo there, the remainder of the vessel would be unaffected. Battle stations were obviously stressful. I ran a series of tests to see how this situation affected the men. I didn't find one case of elevated blood pressure—which suggests that acute stress, when short-lived, is not the cause of hypertension.

However, some studies suggest that people subjected to repeated episodes of stress may be vulnerable. More than twenty years ago, a study of air traffic controllers found that high levels of hypertension were linked to periodic increases in air traffic. The study indicated that hypertension can be produced by acute stress if it occurs repeatedly over a long time.

In a study conducted by Dr. Kathleen Light of the University of North Carolina, it was found that the reaction of a young adult's heart to stress can help predict his risk of high blood pressure later in life. The study demonstrated that men aged 18 to 22 who had at least one parent with hypertension, and had a high response to stress themselves, were more at risk of elevated blood pressure than a control group, who had a low response to stress.

The Role of Stress in Hypertension

What does this mean about stress and the onset of hypertension? From the medical literature as well as my own experience I believe the following to be true:

- Stress may cause hypertension in anyone who is stress-sensitive or who has a predetermined mechanism that responds to stress (or to repeated stress) by developing persistently high blood pressure.
- Added outside stress worsens the condition of hypertensives. Stress will cause high blood pressure to worsen; it then speeds the onset of related complications.

- People predisposed to internally induced stress will develop high blood pressure even if no external stress exists.

- From this, we can draw the following equations about the potential patterns of hypertension:

   Stress-sensitive individual + stress = hypertension

   Hypertensive person + stress = more severe hypertension and complications

   Internally stressed personality + routine life problems = hypertension

CHOLESTEROL AND STRESS

About 40 percent of people with high blood pressure also have high cholesterol levels; stress may be part of this relationship. People with high cholesterol levels had a steep rise in their blood pressure when given a mental stress test; people with normal cholesterol levels had only a modest blood pressure increase.

Stress is a part of life. How you deal with it makes all the difference. It can be toxic, or it can be an inspiration and spur you on to find a better way of life.

The Value of Relaxation Techniques

There are various types of rest therapy, meditation, and mind-body techniques. Rest and relaxation is a way of helping yourself, no matter what technique you use.

In "Elegy Written in a Country Churchyard," the poet Thomas Gray said: "The paths of glory lead but to the grave." For me, this line has served

---

Discrimination Is Stressful

Recent studies suggest that stress caused by discrimination may play a major role in the high rate of hypertension in African-Americans. In one study, those who experienced discrimination but did not report it suffered higher blood pressure more often than those who challenged the discrimination.

as a reminder of the shortness of life. It is something that I have kept in my mind's eye over the years, and it has become my mantra for relaxing. Probably you too have some phrase that can restore your life perspective. (Note: *Mantra* is a Hindu word for an invocation or incantation.)

Find a relaxation technique or a meaningful and calming bit of wisdom that strikes you as very true. You might even want to make it into a sign, and keep in front of you as a reminder; even if you don't, you can try to keep it in the forefront of your mind at all times.

Hobbies offer a wonderful method of relaxation. Many people find painting or drawing or playing a musical instrument excellent ways to unwind. These artistic endeavors need have no other goal than simple enjoyment. Other people find activities like birdwatching a good means of relaxation. The potential avenues of relaxation are numerous. Don't take a passive approach to the problem but rather make positive steps toward developing this means of self-help. It takes only a little time and effort to determine what you like and how you can go about meeting your relaxation requirements.

These techniques have been found to be especially helpful in countering stress. But don't forget you need some stress in your life. Does that surprise you? Perhaps it does, but it is true. Without stress, life would be dull and unexciting. Stress adds novelty, challenge, and opportunity to life. Too much stress, however, can seriously affect your physical and mental well-being. A major challenge in this stress-filled world of today is to make the stress in your life work for you.

Handling Stress

When you face stress it is important to recognize and deal with it. Here are some suggestions for ways to handle stress. As you begin to understand more about how stress affects you as an individual, you will come up with your own ideas of helping to ease the tensions.

Rest and relax: Basic to the treatment and prevention of hypertension is enough rest. It can be physical, emotional, or mental rest, and for most people it must be all three.

Physical activity: The fight-or-flight syndrome means your body is readying itself for running and punching. Running, walking, playing tennis, or working in your garden are some of the adrenaline-burning activities you might try. Physical exercise will relieve that tense feeling and turn the frowns into smiles. Your body and your mind work together.

Share your stress: It helps to talk to someone about your concerns and worries. Perhaps a friend, family member, teacher, or counselor can help you see your problem in a different light. If you feel your problem is serious, you might seek professional help from a psychologist, psychiatrist, social worker, or mental health counselor. Knowing when to ask for help may avoid more serious problems later.

Know your limits: If a problem is beyond your control and cannot be changed at the moment, don't fight the situation. Learn to accept a reality. Don't try to do the impossible. At another time you may be able to change the situation.

Melodic medicine: Music therapy professionals think that music may help to lower blood pressure. Studies suggest that it will soothe you, and transport your thoughts away from any worries. Slow, predictable, and rhythmic music seems to work best. Dancing can also relieve stress; dancing involves both physical activity and soothing or stimulating sounds. Rhythmic movement has been demonstrated to be clinically effective for decreasing bodily tension, reducing chronic pain, and enhancing circulatory and respiratory functions. It also increases a feeling of well-being. And as a form of exercise, it provides all those benefits as well.

Develop a healthy lifestyle: Regular exercise, a healthy diet, and adequate rest are essential to maintaining mental and physical health. Try to surround yourself with people and activities that give you a feeling of control and competence. Are you good at needlework, baking, or woodworking, or even an expert housecleaner? If so, spend more time doing those things that are enjoyable and that you're good at. A hobby is a great stress-reliever.

Make time for fun: Schedule time for both work and recreation. Play can be just as important to your well-being as work; you need a break from your daily routine. Doing something new and even silly may be fun and will help relieve stress.

Be a participant: One way to keep from getting bored, sad, and lonely is to get involved. Instead of feeling sorry for yourself, become a participant. Offer your services to neighborhood or volunteer organizations. Help yourself by helping others. You will be on your way to making new friends and enjoying new activities.

Check off your tasks: Trying to take care of everything at once can seem overwhelming; as a result, you may not accomplish anything and may become even more stressed. Instead, make a list of your tasks, then do them one at a time, giving priority to important tasks and checking them off as they're completed. This will give you a feeling of accomplishment—a great stress reducer.

Must you always be right? Do other people upset you, particularly when they don't do things your way or agree with your opinions? Try cooperation instead of confrontation; it's better than fighting and always needing to be right. A little give-and-take on both sides will reduce the strain and make you both feel more comfortable.

Giggles are good: Laughter is a coordinated arrangement of over a dozen facial muscles propelled by changes in normal breathing. It increases the amount of oxygen that is carried by your blood, and relaxes muscles throughout the face, neck, and body. Laughter also increases blood circulation, which also reduces the risk of blood clots, some types of heart attacks, and strokes. It also seems to improve memory.

It's okay to cry: Crying isn't a form of weakness. Many physicians think it has therapeutic value. Crying can bring relief to your anxiety, and it might even prevent a headache or other physical pain. Take some deep breaths; shallow, nervous breaths can make you hyperventilate and become dizzy; long, deep breathing can release tension.

Create a calming mental scene: A quiet country scene painted mentally, or on canvas, can take you out of the turmoil of a stressful situation. Change the scene by reading a book or playing beautiful music to create a sense of peace and tranquillity. Some people find that staying with their calming scene for about ten minutes works best.

Pet a pet: In a study of elderly patients, pet owners reported fewer doctor visits over a year than those who didn't own pets. Studies indicate that touching, stroking, and cuddling pets reduces a person's heart rate and blood pressure.

Don't self-medicate: Although you can use prescription or over-the-counter medications to relieve stress temporarily, they do not remove the

Pet Magic

Dogs and cats head the list of animals prescribed for pet therapy. Psychologists often write "pet prescriptions." Researchers have identified several ways in which pets help increase their owner's resistance to disease. Pets:

- are companions
- are a source of constancy
- make us laugh and play
- are comfortable and soothing to touch
- give us something to care for
- make us feel safe and secure
- help us get exercise
- provide unconditional love

conditions that caused the stress. Medications, in fact, may be habit-forming and also may reduce your efficiency, thus creating more stress than they take away. They should be taken only on the advice of your doctor.

Down with the decibels: According to researchers at the Department of Public Health and Industrial Hygiene of Kaohsiung Medical College in Japan, shipyard workers who were exposed to noises over 85 decibels (about as loud as a chainsaw) were twice as likely to have high blood pressure as those who worked in a quieter environment.

Avoid environmental stress: Our environment can carry stressors: Food contamination, water and air pollution, microbes, bacteria, and viruses are all around us and within us. Many of us suffer from allergies and are sensitive to certain foods, odors, and smoke. Work toward keeping your neighborhood clean and free of environmental stress.

The Art of Relaxation

The best way to avoid stress is to learn how to relax. Many people try to relax at the same pace that they continue other parts of their lives. That of course won't work, so for a while, tune out your worries about time, pro-

> ### Stress-Fighting Foods
>
> According to researchers at the University of Waterloo, Ontario, Canada, a diet high in omega-3 fatty acids may be helpful in lowering stress. Many people also take antistress nutritional supplements such as multivitamins, vitamin C, calcium, potassium, and magnesium. Tryptophan, which is found in milk, turkey breast meat, walnuts, chickpeas, and wheat germ, has been used to fight insomnia, and in low doses it may be a stress reducer at well.

ductivity, and doing everything right. Find activities that give you pleasure and that are good for your mental and physical well-being. Focus on relaxation, enjoyment, and health. If the stress in your life still seems insurmountable, you may find it beneficial to see a mental health professional.

RELAX AT WORK

You need not lie down to rest. You can rest by developing a system for relaxing. Consider your lunch hour. Divide the time: half for eating your lunch and half for relaxing. The relaxation can be as simple as walking around your company building or sitting on a bench. Enjoy the day—rain or shine, nature is relaxing. Whatever you do, put all your work problems and any other problems out of your mind.

As a result of the advances in electronics, the line between office and home has blurred. I, like many, tried to leave my office problems in the office and relax when I got home. Now one can receive faxes and e-mail twenty-four hours a day. Many of us have lost the ability to turn off the work at home, and as a result our arteries are forced to be in a state of stress—all the time.

You should become aware of the sensation of actual relaxation in your muscles during this resting time. When you are at a stressful meeting (boredom is also stressful), sitting comfortably and breathing deeply will help you relax and be alert at the same time. If you learn to relax, you will help decrease the tension in your system, which in turn will help lower blood pressure.

Start doing this relaxation process for a few minutes at first, then increase the time to ten minutes, then longer. Arrange your files in an inconvenient way so you must get up and move to check a file. Arrange your computer terminal so that you do not have to crane your neck to see the screen. Once you have learned to relax totally, you should increase the frequency of these relaxation periods. On weekends or when you're not working, set aside time after each meal for positive relaxation.

RELAX AT HOME

This system of resting should not be limited to the workday. Sleep is the most basic rest of all, and it is important to use the period of time before going to bed to establish a rest pattern. "Home hydrotherapy" is an ideal way to start. Get into a bathtub filled with warm (not hot) water, and soak for fifteen minutes. Let your muscles relax; if you have been on your feet all day, gently massage your leg muscles to help them relax. (Note: Spending too long in a hot tub is not recommended for people with high blood pressure or heart disease.)

When you get into bed, stretch out full length and get into a comfortable position. Then, concentrating on nothing but your body, start with your head and work downward, relaxing each group of muscles as you progress. Moving down your body, relax your upper arm muscles, then your forearms, then your hands, your thigh muscles, your leg muscles, and your feet.

During this process, work on your mind as well as your body. Clear your mind of any stressful thoughts. In fact, if you think of something very pleasant, you will discover that it helps you relax. You might find music a helpful adjunct to this relaxation technique, but it should be soft music, not anything distracting. Many people have no problem falling asleep but find they wake up after a few hours and are not able to get back to sleep. Fortunately, you can rest without sleeping. Many experts say you should get up, listen to the radio, get on the Internet, or do some other quiet activity.

PROGRESSIVE MUSCLE RELAXATION (PMR)

Stress affects both your mind and body. And you can use body relaxation to fight mental or emotional stress. Relaxing various muscle groups seems to relax the blood flow to these areas. Progressive muscle relaxation involves tensing (stressing) and releasing muscle groups one at a time. Work all your muscle groups, one after another: scalp, face, neck, shoulders, arms, hands, abdomen, back, buttocks, thighs, calves, ankles, and feet.

For example, place your thumbs behind your ears and spread your fingers on top of your head; make a circle in your scalp while moving it slightly. Scrunch your shoulders and then let them go limp. Notice how your muscles feel. Rotate your ankles, curl your toes, and continue until every part of your body has been tensed and relaxed. It will take just a few moments—and leave you relaxed.

A High Blood Pressure Self-Help Technique

If you already have high blood pressure, there is a self-help technique you should know about. First, learn how to take and record your blood pressure. Next, schedule a program of rest at any time you wish during the day or in the evening. You select the time that you are going to rest, and before you start, check your blood pressure; check it again after the rest period is over.

In both instances, be sure to check it in the same manner. If, for example, you were sitting in a chair when you took your blood pressure before your rest, you should be in this position when you take it after resting. By keeping track of your pressure before and after, you can see how helpful these rest periods are for you.

Continue to concentrate on relaxing and on thinking relaxing thoughts. Try increasing your rest periods to see if that helps control your blood pressure. You will see how relaxing and reducing stress helps bring your blood pressure down—and this can be a powerful incentive to reducing stress throughout your day.

There are many other ways to incorporate rest and relaxation periods into your life. Programs that teach or encourage sports, group exercise, and

Stretching and Breathing Exercises

Stretch: Besides easing physical tension and increasing mobility, stretching may help you feel more focused and relaxed. Reach your arms and fingertips to the sky; let your head fall forward; rotate your head, relaxing your shoulders. If you can, get on all fours, arch your back, stretch each leg and each arm. Don't worry about how you look . . . pretend you are a cat.

Breathe: Take slow, deep breaths through your nose. Open your mouth very slightly; let your jaw hang a bit. With your mouth open, blow out air slowly and lightly as if you were blowing out a candle. Avoid short, shallow breathing.

walking groups are in many communities, and many are free. A friend who is in her late sixties attends a tap-dance class. She told me that members of her class range from 8 to 80 years of age. They all have to concentrate to be sure to keep their tapping sound as part of the group. She said not only is it fun, but it's the best stress reliever she has found.

Do whatever works best for you to reduce stress in your life. Your blood pressure will thank you.

CHAPTER 26

Complementary (Alternative) Therapies for Hypertension

There have been dramatic and wonderful changes in medicine during the past few decades. Perhaps the greatest recent change has been the acceptance of alternative medicine used in place of, or in conjunction with, standard Western medical treatments. Four out of ten Americans used at least one alternative medical therapy in 1997 according to a landmark study done by Beth Israel/Deaconess Medical Center in Boston. This study estimates that visits to alternative practitioners increased nearly 50 percent between 1990 and 1997. This trend can be traced to many factors. One of the most important is that many of these techniques require few invasive treatments, involve little or no discomfort, and have few side effects. Everyone wonders, though: Do they work?

What Are Alternative Therapies?

The terms *alternative, complementary,* or *unconventional* when applied to medical therapy cover a wide range of health philosophies, approaches, and methods. Some approaches are consistent with physiological principles of Western medicine, while others constitute independent healing systems. Some of these therapies are far outside the realm of accepted Western medical theory and practice but do seem to alleviate symptoms for many millions of people.

In an effort to study these therapies, a classification system has been designed. This is helpful because many of the alternative systems overlap. Just as in Western medicine, it is often effective to use more than one system.

For example, diet and exercise work together and enhance each other. Some alternative systems seem to have more promise in the treatment of HBP than others. Here are examples of some of the ways that alternative medicine has been classified:

Mind-body systems: meditation, imagery, hypnosis, and biofeedback

Alternative medical systems: acupuncture, naturopathy

Lifestyle and disease prevention: integrated approaches using many theories

Biological therapies: herbal cures, fasting, vegetarianism, vitamin therapy

Manipulative and body-based systems: massage, reflexology, acupressure

In 1992, the National Institutes of Health funded several research projects to investigate alternative treatments, and NIH has made efforts to expand its medical horizons. For more information about this trend and the results of the NIH's research, write: Office of Alternative Medicine, NIH, 6120 Executive Boulevard, EPS Suite 450, Rockville, MD 20892-9904.

Selecting an Alternative Therapy

Before doing anything, you should know that alternative therapies are not always harmless. They run the gamut in terms of their potential for harm, though many are safe. It is important to examine alternative treatments. Here are some guidelines to follow before selecting an alternative therapy:

* Check with your doctor. Always begin by getting a medical diagnosis from a physician. If you decide to try a nonmainstream medical therapy, continue seeing your physician and discuss all treatments with him or her. A competent management of hypertension may require experts in both conventional and alternative therapies.

* Get objective information. Don't rely on people who are promoting the approach, books and magazine articles or the Internet, or some friend who had a good experience. Speak with as many people as you can who have gone through the treatment, and ask about the disadvantages as

well as the advantages. Also ask about the costs, results, and over what time span results can be expected.

* Inquire about the training and expertise of the person administering the treatment (for example, their certification or license to practice in their field). If you still are uncertain, verify the information. Look for a provider who is easy to talk to; you should feel comfortable asking questions. If the methods are too mysterious to understand, or the practitioner is reticent about answering your questions, it is best to avoid that technique.

Mind-Body Therapies and High Blood Pressure

The mind-body connection has long been recognized in standard medicine. The best practitioners have always treated the whole person, not just the disease and its symptoms. For instance, the use of meditation has been accepted practice in reducing stress. It has particular impact on vascular problems. Some mind-body techniques also aim to stimulate the body's immune system and natural defenses rather than only attack germs, viruses, and bacteria.

Awareness of the mind-body connection can often help a patient approach his hypertension in different and insightful ways. There is a distinction between curing and healing: Until recently, "curing" has been the province of the physician, and "healing" the activity of the patient. As with the focus of medicine in the past dozen years, the mind-body connection gives respect and encouragement to both strategies in the improvement of health and well-being.

The placebo response is one of the most widely known examples of mind-body interaction. But surprisingly, it is also one of the most neglected assets in the arsenal of treatments. The placebo response relies heavily on the relationship between doctor and patient. There is a need to provide further medical training on its use and understanding. The mind-body connection is, more and more, becoming part of standard Western medicine. The therapeutic potential of spirituality, prayer, and religion (organized and personal), neglected until recently, is now also being studied in many medical universities. The ability of most people to actually effect changes in their internal systems has been well documented by many physicians throughout medical history. Specific mind-body interventions that may help in managing hypertension include counseling, support groups, and meditation:

Counseling: Talking to and listening to patients has always been part of the clinical physician's examination. What the patient doesn't say, as well as what he or she does say, can lead to a better diagnosis.

Support groups: These can have a powerful positive effect in a wide variety of physical illnesses, including heart disease, high blood pressure, and stroke. Support groups have many benefits. They help members form empowering bonds with each other. Support groups also validate any feelings of depression or frustration that people who are working through problems usually have. Group interaction also prevents people from feeling isolated, and groups are low-cost or free.

Meditation: During the past three decades in the West, meditation has been explored as a way of reducing stress on both mind and body and is often recommended as a way of reducing high blood pressure. In the 1960s the Maharishi Mahesh Yogi, a guru, brought a simplified form of yoga to the West; he called his method Transcendental Meditation (TM). (The terms *TM* and *meditation* are used here interchangeably.) This self-directed practice was designed to relax the body and calm the mind. Practitioners of meditation have been observed to have a remarkable capacity to control certain mechanisms of the autonomic nervous system, the part of the nervous system that controls involuntary muscles, such as the heart. Most meditative techniques have come to the West from Eastern religious practices, particularly those of India, China, and Japan. They have been associated with ancient spiritual techniques used in Zen Buddhism and yoga. Meditation techniques can be found in many cultures throughout the world.

HOW TO MEDITATE

Check your blood pressure before and after you meditate, so you can evaluate the success of meditation. Find a quiet, comfortable place at a quiet, unhurried time of the day. Morning and early evening are preferred by many people. Avoid meditating right before or after meals, as hunger and digestion will interfere with the meditative process. Meditating requires stillness and concentration.

Meditation involves sitting in a comfortable position and clearing your mind of stressful thoughts. (Note: Lying down is not suggested for medita-

---

A Validated Program

Transcendental meditation seems to banish stress, and it has several other uses as well. According to the TM program for Delaware County, Pennsylvania, over five hundred scientific research and clinical studies conducted during the past twenty-five years at more than two hundred universities and institutes in thirty countries have shown that meditation may:

- Eliminate accumulated stress from the nervous system
- Provide a natural remedy for stress-related disorders, including insomnia, chronic anxiety, hypertension, addiction, headache, depression, panic attacks, and learning disorders.
- Help in developing self-esteem, self-control, and self-confidence.

---

tion.) You may find that relaxing your hands in your lap, palms up, will help. Place your feet slightly apart on the floor. Concentrate on your breathing; breathe in deeply, and then pause, and release air. Start meditating by softly repeating a soothing sound or word. Repeat your calming sound or word, or focus on a calming scene, for about twenty minutes at each sitting, or as long as it feels comfortable.

MEDITATION STUDIES AND HIGH BLOOD PRESSURE

Meditation lowers blood pressure: Researchers studied 111 men and women with high blood pressure. After three months, meditation significantly lowered systolic blood pressure 10.7 mm Hg and diastolic blood pressure 6.4 mm Hg compared with a control group. The study also found that the program was about twice as effective as progressive muscle relaxation, and produced about twice the reduction in blood pressure commonly found in previous trials of diet and exercise.

Meditation means relief: In a three-month clinical experiment with elderly people dwelling in an inner-city community, meditation lowered systolic and diastolic blood pressure by 10.6 and 5.9 mm HG respectively. A study with the elderly conducted at Harvard University found similar blood pressure changes.

Other studies have found that regular meditation can also reduce the need for health care, increase longevity and quality of life, reduce chronic pain, reduce anxiety, lower serum cholesterol level, reduce substance abuse, reduce post-traumatic stress syndrome in war veterans, and dissipate anger and stress.

Other Mind-Body Connections

Meditation is only one of the ways you can train yourself to break the stress cycle. Several other ways are described briefly below. If you find them more useful, you can learn more about them. Perhaps one may seem more appealing to you or can be used more conveniently. They have all been used with varying degrees of success.

Imagery (Visualization): This is a mental process using various procedures. It is often defined as creating any thought which conjures up any sensory reaction. For example: Think of licking an ice-cold ice cream. Imagine the way it feels on your tongue. Visualize the way it melts. Imagery has been tested to alleviate nausea and to relieve stress; it has also been used for pain control and for several diseases including diabetes. It is most often used to train people to mobilize their immune systems.

Breathing: Slow exhaling is just as important as slow inhaling. If you purposefully breathe in a slow, rhythmic way for about five minutes a day, it can be relaxing and may lower your blood pressure and pulse rate.

Hypnosis: Modern hypnosis began in the eighteenth century. In the past fifty years, hypnosis has been used to fight addictions and control pain. However, there are few verifiable studies to show any links between hypnosis and HBP.

Yoga: This is a system of ethical precepts and dietary prescriptions combined with physical exercise. To date, thousands of research studies have been undertaken and have shown that with yoga a person can learn to control such physiological functions as blood pressure, heart rate, and breathing.

Spiritual healing: Prayer and mental/spiritual techniques often require the healer to enter a prayerful, altered state of consciousness. In other methods, holding hands, chanting, breathing smoke, whirling, or repeating sounds or chants or motions can place a person in an altered state.

In addition to preventing or managing hypertension, these therapies, and others like them, provide people with the opportunity to be involved with their own care. Just as a low-salt, low-cholesterol diet and exercise are under each person's control, many of the techniques of mind-body therapies are also within a person's control.

Many patients believe their doctor or medical system is too technical and impersonal and too eager to prescribe chemical solutions (pills or medications). The mind-body approach is potentially corrective of some of these complaints. If appropriately selected and wisely used, mind-body techniques such as biofeedback (discussed in the next chapter) and meditation can provide wonderful results.

CHAPTER 27

Biofeedback: Training Your Body to Reduce Hypertension

The term *biofeedback* describes a method used to control your internal physiological reactions, such as muscle tension and blood flow. Biofeedback trains your mind to "feed back" suggestions into your body systems. It gives you a way to change internal automatic patterns to new patterns that are less stressful and healthier for you. Biofeedback has been demonstrated to slow heart rate and reduce blood pressure. Since hypertension is often a stress-related condition, biofeedback control of stress also has value in high blood pressure treatment. And there is a bonus: People who master biofeedback often experience a renewed sense of physical and mental well-being.

How Biofeedback Works

Biofeedback techniques use electronic equipment to identify the various electrical patterns that are produced within the body as a result of muscle contractions, heartbeat, and brain waves. It allows you to observe these ordinarily unseen and silent reflex patterns as patterns of light and sound. As the electrical pattern within the body increases, the sound gets louder, and as the electrical pattern decreases, the sound, too, decreases. The person using biofeedback learns to control body function by creating changes in the light patterns or sounds. This control of body function, as reflected through the light signals on the screen and beeping sounds, usually is attained by learning how to achieve relaxation.

Biofeedback gives us information about our bodies just as using a thermometer gives us information about body temperature. Moving graphs on a computer screen and sound tones display and measure changes in the body systems, such as muscle tension. To understand how this works, compare the body system's regulation to the heat and air-conditioning systems in a large building. When the outside temperature rises, the air-conditioning goes on. When the temperature falls, the heat goes on. The thermostat that regulates the temperature is really a feedback system that responds to temperature changes.

Biofeedback is a way to recognize your body's responses to thoughts, but it requires concentration and practice. Through practice, we become familiar with our own normal patterns and learn how to change these patterns. It is "mind over blood pressure." Trying to change internal physiological activity without biofeedback is like playing tennis in the dark—you cannot see where the ball goes or how well you are doing. Through biofeedback instruments, we know when we are changing our pattern and in which direction. Once you master the technique, the biofeedback instrumentation is no longer needed.

Instruments Used in Feedback

Biofeedback uses a sensitive instrument designed to measure certain physical processes. The biofeedback instrument is connected to your skin and underlying muscles with sensors. The sensors, which do not hurt or irritate you, are placed on the skin. These sensors amplify and convert the physical response of the blood supply and muscles to information in the form of light and sound. This feedback is used as a baseline to help you practice a variety of procedures to reduce muscle tension The electronic machine is like a mirror that reflects what is going on inside rather than on the surface. The equipment commonly used to identify and study various body activities includes:

Electromyography (EMG): The electromyograph measures the electrical activity of muscles using sensors placed on the skin over muscles. The instrument is an electrosensory recording system that picks up the minute electrical signals emitted by the muscles as they contract. An electrode or sensor is used to absorb the signal; it is transformed and amplified so it can be seen on a screen and heard in the form of popping sounds. The greater the degree of activity within the muscle the more sound is produced.

In this way the instrument feeds back information to the individual so he or she can learn to control the degree of muscular activity. Initially, to learn the variables of control, patients tighten their muscles and move them. Later they work on relaxing these muscles.

EMG has been used as a tool in the treatment and management of stress and for general relaxation training. It is often used for the treatment of tension headache, bruxism (teeth grinding during sleep), pain, spasm, and other muscular dysfunction due to stroke or congenital disorders.

Thermal (blood flow) feedback: When the small vessels in the skin dilate, blood flow and temperature of the skin increase; when vessels constrict, blood flow and temperature decrease. (Finger temperature is a useful tool in thermal feedback training.) Blood flow feedback is also used in the treatment of vascular disorders such as migraine headache, Raynaud's disease, essential hypertension, and vascular complication of diabetes.

Electrodermal feedback: The electrodermal response (EDR) feedback instruments measure skin conductively from the fingers and palms. Skin is very sensitive to emotions. EDR feedback has been used in the treatment of excessive sweating (hyperhidrosis) and related skin conditions and for relaxation training.

Brain wave feedback: The electroencephalograph (EEG) uses sensors placed on the scalp. Applications for EEG feedback are still being studied; it is now often used in sleep clinics.

Special applications: Other instruments have been developed to facilitate self-regulation in a variety of stress-related and organic disorders such as irregular heartbeats.

How to Use Biofeedback

An example of how this relaxation training works appears in the following excerpt from *From the Inside Out: A Self-Teaching and Laboratory Manual for Biofeedback,* by Erik Pepper and Elizabeth Ann Williams. "Get in a comfortable position. Minimally tighten your right fist so that you feel only the smallest amount of tension. Hold it at this level. Be sure you continue to

> ### Relaxation Studies
>
> Caracas, Venezuela: A study shows that people who learned biofeedback had a significant reduction in systolic and diastolic values. In a six-month follow-up, the group studied still showed lowered pressure.
>
> Toledo, Ohio: One hundred and one patients, diagnosed with hypertension, were examined for the effects of biofeedback on blood pressure: Treatment yielded short-term success; other significant short-term changes included reduction of both muscle tension and anxiety.

breathe. . . . Now let go and relax. . . . Observe the difference in feeling between the right and left arm and fist. Now minimally tighten your left fist. Hold this level so that you just feel the tightening. . . . Let go and relax. Let the relaxation spread through the arms and the rest of the body."

One of my patients told me that she developed her ability to use biofeedback by thinking of boiled eggs. She used feedback to keep her fingers warm when she had to wait for a bus that didn't come—during a snowstorm. She thinks of taking the boiled eggs from the hot cooking water. Her fingers touch each egg and feel warm as she pretends to take it from the very hot water. Surprisingly, she said that her fingers became very much warmer. She believes she was conducting her blood flow to her fingers through the power of her mind—biofeedback.

The Electroencephalograph— The Brain Wave Machine

One of the most important instruments used in biofeedback is the electroencephalograph (EEG). Often called the brain wave machine, it records in graphic tracings the minute electrical waves produced by the brain cells as they function. It is widely used in medical practice as a diagnostic tool because it can identify abnormal wave patterns associated with brain diseases, when it is used in conjunction with MRIs and other imaging systems. The waves are received by an electrode or sensor placed on the scalp and are magnified before being printed out in patterns on a moving tape. These wave patterns were first described in 1929 by a German physiologist who named them alpha, beta, delta, and theta after letters of the Greek alphabet.

BRAIN WAVES

Alpha: These waves are signals that the mind (brain) is turned inward and, although still alert, is relaxed.

Beta: These waves show that attention is focused on solving a problem or some aspect of the outside world; beta waves also are seen during emotional periods.

Delta: These waves are emitted by the brain during sleep.

Theta: These waves occur when a person is drowsy but not asleep. Images are formed within the brain; some people feel their creativity is stimulated during this time.

THE IMPORTANCE OF ALPHA WAVES

Alpha waves are of special interest in biofeedback. Alpha waves are slow, rhythmic, and occur in cycles that average about ten per second. Biofeedback is directed toward reducing both internal and external stress, and the alpha waves are the measure of the state of relaxation that must be achieved to find relief from stress. However, this relationship is not as simple as it might seem. Non-stress-related matters can interfere with the alpha waves. Some experts believe alpha waves are easily altered and can even be increased when the subject's eyes are open rather than closed.

Does Biofeedback Really Work?

Does biofeedback work in cases of stress-related problems? Its proponents believe it is of value for any mental or physical symptoms with stress-related components. Critical evaluation of this concept is difficult to produce. It is a vast field, and control studies are difficult to organize, but positive evaluations are in the news from time to time.

It seems clear that certain people, in certain situations, would be greatly aided by the use of any relaxation technique. I can think of some patients who are characteristic type A personalities—tense, driven to succeed, and anxiety-prone. For these people, biofeedback therapy could be of value. The typical case often cited in the biofeedback literature involves a woman with tension headaches who obtains substantial or total headache relief by learning to control the muscle tensions of her body, particularly the muscles in the areas about the neck and head.

For some with hypertension, stress-controlled biofeedback is possible, but how well it works depends on the individual. As we have seen, hypertension usually develops from many causes, and the disorder in any person may result from more than one cause. However, biofeedback can help patients in whom hypertension is triggered by stress.

Biofeedback and Hypertension

Exactly what value does biofeedback have in the treatment of hypertension? The answer is not simple. As soon as it was brought into use, it was seized upon by faddists and nonscientific workers who felt it would answer almost every problem. It cannot. It is appealing to think that you can learn to control your internal environment (body systems) and modify reflex actions.

STUDIES SHOW BIOFEEDBACK CAN HELP

When we experience stress certain physiological changes take place. One of them is increased activity in the sympathetic nervous system, which results in constrictions in our blood vessels. The vessels in our fingers are very sensitive to stress (constriction) and to relaxation (dilation). When these blood vessels in our hands and feet are constricted, blood is diverted away from those extremities, resulting in cold fingers and higher blood pressure.

In 1995, research demonstrated that you can undo this cold-fingered rise in pressure. Biofeedback monitoring and learning to warm fingers

Jan Lowers Her Blood Pressure Using Biofeedback

Jan began to have severe headaches soon after her thirtieth birthday; when they began interfering with her demanding job, she sought medical advice. After a series of tests it was found that Jan had essential hypertension. Jan's physician suggested she try to find ways to alleviate the tension caused by her job with biofeedback; the results were gratifying. When away from work, Jan learned to focus her thinking and to leave her office problems in the office. Daily biofeedback exercises helped lower her blood pressure and bring relief from the headaches. Jan's mind-body therapy was all that was needed.

through stress management can help reduce sympathetic nervous system activity and relieve the constricted finger and toe blood vessels, and thus lower blood pressure.

In another study, conducted several years ago, an attempt was made to teach people to control their blood pressure via biofeedback. A blood pressure device was used so that each person could monitor his or her pressure. The subjects tried to raise their pressure when a green light went on and tried to reduce it when a red light went on; when they were successful, a yellow light went on.

Using this method, some people were able to lower their systolic pressure from an average of 141 mm Hg to an average of 125 mm Hg at home using techniques learned in the laboratory. The conclusion of this study was that biofeedback can temporarily lower blood pressure in patients with mild hypertension.

Finding a Biofeedback Therapist

Biofeedback therapists are health professionals who use biofeedback training in their work. Many psychologists, social workers, nurses, physical therapists, and other health care professionals have been trained to use biofeedback. Health care workers who do not have a professional degree may be trained and work under the supervision of a licensed practitioner. The Biofeedback Certification Institute of America (BCIA) certifies therapists through a national examination.

The length of your biofeedback treatment varies; sometimes a series of treatments will take only eight to ten sessions. Because relaxation and stress management are learned skills, practice will lead to improvement; on the other hand, treatment may end before all the symptoms are managed. The cost will vary with clinic or therapist and the number of sessions needed. Note: Biofeedback is covered by many health insurance groups. Consult your insurance company before you start treatments.

To locate a biofeedback therapist, begin with the yellow pages in the telephone book; look under "Biofeedback" or "Psychologists." You can also write for a list of certified practitioners in your area to the Biofeedback Certification Institute of America at 10200 West 44th Avenue, Suite 304, Wheat Ridge, CO 80033; 303-420-2902. If you want a brochure to learn more about biofeedback, enclose a stamped, self-addressed envelope.

Some Final Words on the Efficacy of Biofeedback

A study group of the American College of Physicians evaluated the use of biofeedback in the treatment of hypertension and came to the following conclusions:

- Biofeedback cannot be recommended as first-line treatment for essential hypertension. It is suggested that the initial nondrug approach to the problem should be lifestyle counseling in such areas as weight reduction, regular exercise, reduction of salt intake, and quitting smoking. (Interestingly, this group failed to mention a reduction in alcohol intake.)

- Biofeedback may be a useful adjunct in reducing medication requirements for patients with mild hypertension or for those who suffer adverse reactions to medication. As is the case with medication or other antihypertensive therapies, the use of biofeedback requires keeping track of your blood pressure.

- Biofeedback is no more effective than other therapies such as yoga, meditation, and various other self-relaxation techniques.

- Further trials are recommended with large groups of people and long-term follow-up, including extensive monitoring of daily blood pressure levels, to better judge the effects of biofeedback. Many issues about the method of treatment need to be resolved, and in particular, an attempt should be made to identify patients who would be most likely to benefit from biofeedback and other nonmedicinal treatments.

MY OWN CONCLUSIONS

My impression is that there is value in the therapy, but there is difficulty evaluating the real results. Medical practice uses many therapies that aid only a fraction of the people being treated. If we knew how to select those people who would benefit from a specific therapy, many disappointments would be averted. My approach is to try this therapy and then evaluate the results on a patient-by-patient basis. If biofeedback helps, excellent. If not, the patient suffers no ill effects. Obviously, if there is any indication of a rise in blood pressure during biofeedback, it should be stopped immediately and not be used.

In considering the value of biofeedback training in controlling hypertension, the diversity of the factors that cause high blood pressure must be considered; there may be a place for biofeedback in the treatment of some patients. From my personal experience with this type of therapy, I am convinced that the ability to learn to relax can have very positive results, even if the actual drop in blood pressure is small.

Many people have found relief through biofeedback. But as always, adherence to a low-sodium diet, exercise, and other strategies is important, with or without biofeedback or other relaxation techniques.

CHAPTER 28

Folk Medicine and Other Traditions

Worldwide, only about 10 to 30 percent of the health care is delivered using conventional Western medical theory. The remaining 70 to 90 percent of people are treated via self-care, according to folk beliefs, or by care given in an organized health care system based on non-Western (alternative) traditions.

In recent years, as commerce, culture, and the Internet have encouraged us to become more international in outlook, health care and theories from other cultures have been introduced into the United States. There are now many professional health care providers who have been trained in the traditions of Asian medicine, acupuncture, ayurvedic medicine, homeopathy, native beliefs, naturopathy, and environmental medicine. These systems, many of which have professional health care practitioners, have formal philosophies and practitioners who undergo formal training. I have met many of them, and they are dedicated to the health and well-being of their patients. Below are some of the alternative systems of medical practice that seem most relevant to HBP and are being studied by the National Institutes of Health.

Traditional Asian Medicine

Asian (or Oriental, as it is commonly called) medicine, as practiced in China, is a set of systematic techniques and methods including acupuncture, herbal medicine, acupressure, qi gong, and massage. Most striking is its emphasis on diagnosing disturbances of qi (vital energy).

Tai Chi Lowers Blood Pressure

In April of 1998, a seminar at Johns Hopkins University of Medicine discussed a study of more than sixty men and women aged 60 and older that indicated those using the tai chi system of meditative movements had systolic blood pressure drops nearly equal to those of a group who were involved in aerobic exercise. The conclusion was that for elderly, sedentary people, getting up and doing even some slow movement was associated with a reduction in high blood pressure.

In the United States, the professional practitioner's base for Oriental medicine is organized around acupuncturist practitioners and the use of Asian medicines. Traditional Oriental herbal medicine and formulas have been studied for their therapeutic value in alleviating hypertension as well as many other long-term syndromes, acquired immunodeficiency syndrome (AIDS), and certain cancers.

ACUPUNCTURE

Acupuncture involves stimulating specific points in the body for therapeutic purposes. Puncturing the skin with a very thin needle is the usual method, but practitioners also use heat, pressure, friction, suction, or impulses of electromagnetic energy to stimulate the points. In the last forty years it has become well known and reasonably available. About three thousand conventionally trained U.S. physicians have taken courses so that they could incorporate acupuncture in their medical practice. It is particularly useful in resolving physical problems related to tension and stress, migraine headaches, and emotional conditions.

The explanation is that channels of energy run in regular patterns through the body and over its surface. These energy channels, called meridians, are like rivers flowing through the body irrigating and nourishing the tissues. Acupuncturists maintain that these rivers can become blocked at certain points and that the acupuncture needles clear these obstructions. The modern scientific explanation is that needling the acupuncture points stimulates the nervous system to release chemicals in the muscles, spinal cord, and brain.

Do the needles hurt? Acupuncture needles are very thin and solid and are made from stainless steel. The point is smooth (not hollow, as with a

> ### Demonstrated Use
>
> My experience with acupuncture needles dates back to the time when I was operating at St. Vincent's Hospital in New York City. One of our operating room nurses visited China and brought back a number of acupuncture needles. She demonstrated their use and I found it most interesting. One particular spot was on the web section of the hand between the thumb and first finger. It is used to reduce fever. At this time, I'm not totally convinced, but I remain interested in new—and ancient—ideas.

hypodermic needle) and insertion through the skin is not as painful as injections or blood samples, nor is there as much bruising and skin irritation as with hollow needles.

Extensive research has been done in China studying acupuncture's therapeutic value in reducing hypertension, and according to this research it seems to work. It would be useful to repeat these studies in the United States, assessing a U.S. clinical population according to our research criteria. If you want more information, write the American Academy of Medical Acupuncture, 5820 Wilshire Boulevard, Suite 500, Los Angeles, CA 90036.

AYURVEDA

India's traditional, natural system of medicine has been practiced for more than five thousand years. Ayurvedic theory states that disease begins with imbalance or stress. Lifestyle interventions are a major therapeutic approach. The research is ongoing, and it is focused on the physiological effects of meditative techniques and yoga postures. Published studies have documented reductions in cardiovascular disease risk factors, including blood pressure, cholesterol, and reaction to stress in individuals who practice ayurvedic methods.

Other Alternative/Complementary Systems

The following are other systems, theories, approaches, and ideas. It is too early in the research to tell which may be of use in your efforts to lower blood pressure. What is encouraging is that these ideas give you options in your lifestyle modifications. To me, the recurring efforts of many cultures, from the most ancient Indian and Chinese to modern Western, often take into account the mind-body connection.

HOMEOPATHIC MEDICINE

Homeopathic remedies are made from naturally occurring plant, animal, or mineral substances, are recognized and regulated by the Food and Drug Administration, and are manufactured by established pharmaceutical companies. Recent clinical trials suggest that homeopathic medicines have a positive effect on allergies and influenza. Nothing is demonstrated thus far on hypertension.

NATUROPATHY

Founded as a formal health care system about a hundred years ago, as practiced today, naturopathic medicine integrates traditional natural therapeutics, including botanical medicine, clinical nutrition, homeopathy, acupuncture, traditional Oriental medicine, hydrotherapy, and manipulative therapy.

Touch and Manipulation

As we've seen, petting a beloved animal lowers blood pressure. Could touch and manipulation with the hands overcome certain diseases? Here are some of the techniques that incorporate this approach:

CHIROPRACTIC SCIENCE

This system focuses on the relationship between the spine and the nervous system. Chiropractic physicians use manual procedures rather than surgical or chemical treatments. They believe that blood pressure is an important indication of internal body conditions. Normal pressure varies with each individual. High or low blood pressure in the chiropractic view may be indicative of abnormal nerve function.

MASSAGE THERAPY

One of the oldest methods in health care practice is the scientific manipulation of the soft body tissues. Primarily the hands are used, but sometimes forearms, elbows, and feet are used as well. These techniques can affect the musculoskeletal, circulatory-lymphatic, and nervous systems. Many patients report feelings of stress-free relaxation and well-being after a massage. Massage therapists are licensed in many states. Here is a list of only some of the types of massage:

Swedish massage: This is the most common style of massage. It is done using the fingers and hands. Oil or powder is rubbed on the bare skin to smooth the therapist's strokes. Swedish massage is used for relaxation and to improve circulation.

Deep tissue massage: Similar to Swedish massage, deep tissue massage uses more pressure.

Shiatsu: This Japanese cousin of acupuncture uses pressure on meridians to open channels.

Reflexology: This is similar to shiatsu, but it's done primarily on the feet. By pressing on certain points, the therapist aims to treat various organs and glands. (Note: I have doubts about this one.)

Reiki: This is a no-pressure massage in which the therapist places hands on specific areas of the body to transfer energy.

From electromagnetic therapy to environmental medicine, new and ancient theories are being investigated. The important thing to remember is that there are some techniques that we now know work very well: exercise, a low-salt/low-fat diet, stress reduction, reduced alcohol consumption, quitting smoking, and adherence to your physician's recommendations. If you find some of these alternative methods interesting, talk with your doctor about them, but don't abandon your present program. For more information about alternative medicine, write to the Office of Alternative Medicine, NIH, 6120 Executive Boulevard, EPS Suite 450, Rockville, MD 20892.

CHAPTER 29

Exercise Combats Hypertension

There is a strategy to lower HBP that is completely natural, is both ancient and modern, and also Western and Oriental, and that is under your control, with proven results, and is inexpensive as well as being available to you right now. It is exercise.

We are coming to recognize the value of regular exercise in combating a wide variety of diseases and disorders. This appears to be as true for hypertension as for several other physical disorders. Any type of physical activity you choose, whether strenuous, such as running or aerobic dancing, or of moderate intensity, such as walking or housecleaning, will increase the number of calories your body uses. The key to a successful exercise program that will control hypertension, and provide the bonus of a reduction of weight, is making physical activity a part of your daily routine.

A number of studies have been conducted to evaluate the effect of exercise on blood pressure and other diseases in people of various ages and with several different diseases and conditions. These studies have shown that regular physical activity can help protect you from the following health problems:

Heart disease and stroke: Daily physical activity can strengthen your heart muscle, lower blood pressure, raise your high-density lipoprotein (HDL, the good cholesterol) and lower low-density lipoprotein (LDL, the bad cholesterol) levels, improve blood flow, and increase your heart and blood vessel capacity.

Non-insulin-dependent diabetes: By reducing body fat, physical activity can help to prevent or control this type of diabetes.

Back pain: By increasing muscle strength and endurance and improving flexibility and posture, regular exercise helps prevent pain.

Osteoporosis: Regular weight-bearing exercise promotes bone formation and may prevent many forms of bone loss. Exercise also improves balance and increases muscle strength, thus lowering the risk of falls.

Depression and mood disorders: Studies on the psychological effects of exercise have found that regular activity can improve the way you feel about yourself. Research also indicates exercise is likely to reduce depression, anxiety, and stress.

Keep all these health benefits in mind when you consider a program of physical activity. It can't be stressed enough: Any amount of physical activity you do is better than none at all.

Exercise for Your Body and Brain

Exercise and sports do two essential things for the body: They burn up calories, and they build muscles. If we did not burn the calories, the food we eat would turn to fat. Adequate physical exercise often results in a decrease in weight, blood pressure, and essential hypertension.

Although most discussions of exercise and sports stress the physical changes and benefits that can be derived, also important is the feeling of well-being. This good feeling is believed to result from an increase in a kind of naturally occurring narcotic in the body called endorphins. Certainly, if essential hypertension has as its basis an element of stress, then an increase in natural body chemicals that contribute to a sense of ease may lessen hypertension. Moreover, it is far easier to watch calories when you are feeling good about yourself than when you are depressed. Susan, a young patient, was an example of this. At 21, Susan had a weight problem that diets only temporarily succeeded in relieving. When she resumed her normal eating routine, she regained any weight she lost. Susan finally solved her weight problem by joining an exercise group at the local Y. Exercising and a daily swim made her feel, in her words, "really good." Susan also noticed that after exercising she felt no need to "pig out." For Susan, the activity resulted in both feeling good and burning off fat.

> ## Exercise Lowers Blood Pressure
>
> *The American Journal of Hypertension,* 1998: Ninety-seven men, all seden-
> tary nonsmokers, 45 years of age and older, were assigned to one of four
> programs:
>
> > aerobic exercise
> >
> > aerobic exercise combined with weight loss
> >
> > weight loss without aerobic exercise
> >
> > sedentary control group
>
> After nine months, researchers found that blood pressure in the control
> group did not change, but those men in the aerobic exercise program had a
> 7 mm Hg drop in systolic blood pressure and 5 mm Hg in diastolic blood
> pressure. The men in the weight loss group also noticed a similar drop in
> pressure. The researchers also found that a combination of aerobic exercise
> and weight loss resulted in better results on many tests.

EXERCISES ARE NOT ALL THE SAME

There are three main types of exercise: isotonic (aerobic), isometric, and
isokinetic.

Isotonic (aerobic) exercise involves the repeated and constant use of
the large muscles of the body. Walking, jogging, swimming, and cycling are
good examples of this kind of exercise.

Isometric exercise, such as weight lifting, produces massive enlargement of the muscles, but it doesn't do much for your cardiovascular system. Avoid exercises that employ movements in which the arms are held
overhead, as these increase blood pressure and heart rate. Not only is it in-
advisable to use these exercises if you have high blood pressure, they may
be dangerous to your health.

Isokinetic exercise is comparatively new. It develops muscular strength
by means of specially designed exercise equipment that provides a resistance equal to the force applied by the person doing the exercise.

Writing in *The Physician and Sports Medicine* in 1992, Barry M. Massie,
M.D., noted, "Aerobic exercise creates a much smaller rise in blood pres-

sure during exertion and is more likely to increase aerobic capacity and improve blood profiles than other exercise strategies. Isokinetic and isotonic resistance training may be implemented only when very light weights are used. Pure isometric exercises are not recommended for hypertensives."

How Does Exercise Alter Blood Pressure?

Any type of exercise causes an immediate rise in blood pressure, but this rise is short-term, lasting only as long as the exercise. The rise in blood pressure follows a physiological pattern, which explains why some exercises are good for you and others are dangerous.

When you exercise, the rise in blood pressure can be high or moderate, depending on the body's response to stress resulting from the demand for energy. The nervous system charges up all the body systems and, in so doing, increases the central body blood pressure. This is done by a special branch of the nervous system, the sympathetic branch, which prepares the body for increased efforts. When you use a muscle for work or exercise, it calls for an increase in blood flow by opening numerous blood vessels. This draws blood from the central system, decreasing the pressure in direct proportion to the pressure accepted by the newly opened blood vessels.

If you use only a few muscles, the decrease in central pressure is slight, and the body pressure can rise quite high. When you use large numbers of muscles, as in swimming, cross-country skiing, or jogging, the newly opened vessels draw off a large volume of blood, reducing the central level. Exercises that use large numbers of muscles are best for the person with essential hypertension. The pressure rises only a little, and the danger of a blood vessel rupture is slight.

When Exercise Is Not Good

People with hypertension secondary to tumors of the adrenal gland, diseases of the thyroid gland, kidney disease, any brain disease, or any disease of the main artery of the body, the aorta, should refrain from exercise that may elevate the blood pressure. Increased pressure can strain the arterial walls, and if there are weak areas, such pressure can rupture the walls. This is what happens when someone has an aneurysm.

Some studies suggest that exercise, and in particular, certain kinds of exercise, is not always beneficial even in those with essential hypertension. I

Medication and Exercise Interactions

Although of course anyone who embarks on an exercise program should check with his physician, this is especially true if you take blood pressure medication.

Beta-blockers are prescribed to lower blood pressure, but when mixed with vigorous exercise, they limit exercise-related improvements in blood lipids. Beta-blockers are less apt to interfere with only low or moderate activity.

If you have hypertension and plan to participate in vigorous activity, then certain forms of calcium channel blockers or angiotensin converting enzyme (ACE) inhibitors may be prescribed by your doctor. Caution should be taken if you are on diuretics and performing high-intensity exercise. High-intensity exercise promotes sweating, and heavy sweating can increase the risk of potassium depletion and dehydration. Note: Before exercising, do not drink caffeinated beverages or use a caffeinated over-the-counter medication, which may increase the heart rate and blood pressure during physical activity.

mention these studies to give a balanced view, although I believe, as a result of my experience, that exercise is of great value to this group.

The key to the use of exercise to control or prevent high blood pressure depends entirely on the correct use of this therapy. The exercises you choose should not be too taxing; they should be increased on a progressive basis and done regularly so there is no sudden or undue strain. Overexertion or too great stress at any one time should always be avoided.

In his 1994 book, *Living a Healthy Life with Chronic Conditions,* Halstead Holman, M.D., lays out some caveats. He suggests that before beginning any conditioning program, check with your physician to make sure your blood pressure is under control. He also warns against exercises that cause you to strain while holding your breath (isometric exercise, weight lifting, and rowing, for example). But he gives a thumbs-up to endurance exercises that rhythmically contract and relax muscles, because they are generally not harmful and may help you lower blood pressure. It would be a good idea to monitor your blood pressure before and after exercise as well.

An Exercise Program Just for You

Prior to any exercise program, complete a medical history with your doctor as well as a physical examination, which should include blood tests and urinalyses. If your history reveals any potential illnesses or if your physical exam reveals any abnormalities, they should be evaluated before you start.

There is an exercise for everyone. Finding the program that is best suited to your needs requires that you evaluate your physical fitness and target some long- and short-term exercise goals. Here are some questions you will want to ask yourself or discuss with your family and physician before you begin your new exercise program:

- How fit are you now? Have you been inactive for several years? If you haven't exercised recently you should start with less strenuous activities and gradually, as you get into better shape, make your routine more challenging. If you are over 50 and have not been active, this is especially true. (Note: The Senior Softball Association says that a fit 70-year-old can have more aerobic capacity than a 25-year-old who lives a sedentary life.)

- Do you like exercising alone or with other people? Do you like to exercise outdoors or indoors? Do you want privacy when you exercise? Team sports often provide a secondary benefit—you can get validation and encouragement from your fellow team members. Outdoor activities offer a variety of scenery and weather but are less convenient than at-home activities.

- Will your exercise or activity strain your budget? Running and tennis can be inexpensive, but skiing and some other sports may involve clothing, equipment, or transportation costs. Many communities provide inexpensive exercise locations; look in the Yellow Pages of your telephone book or call your local municipal office. They will be glad to provide you with information. Start at your level of fitness and keep exercising. Change the activity if one gets boring, or you find some other drawback. There are activities for every level. Most important: Do it.

START SLOWLY WITH A STRETCH

Are you someone who has not exercised at all in the past, or for the past dozen years or so? If you fit this description, start by selecting a routine you can do when you get out of bed in the morning. (These stretches are valuable for everyone to do before exercising.) Once you start, make it a rule that you will do this exercise daily, and don't skip a day. When you get into a pattern of regular exercise you will find it becomes increasingly easier to continue. The beauty of simple exercises is that they require no equipment and not very much space. Start with as many of the following simple routines as you can comfortably do, performing them in sequence if possible:

- Stretch both arms outward and gently rotate them in small circles in a clockwise and then counterclockwise manner. Start with three each way, each day, and increase the number, always at least maintaining the previous day's number.

- Raise your arms over your head and stretch them as far forward and then as far backward as you can before lowering them. Breathe deeply with each stretching action. Fill your lungs as you raise your arms, and slowly let the air out as you lower them. (Do not do this too quickly, since it is possible to hyperventilate, which can cause you to become dizzy.)

- Rotate your head in a complete circle. Stretch your neck muscles by pushing your chin down on your chest. Next, stretch your head back as far as you can. Then stretch to one side and then to the other.

- Try to touch your toes without bending your knees. Do so gently; do not force yourself too far, for it is possible to injure the ligaments in your knees if you press too hard. If you cannot get down all the way, spread your legs farther apart until you can touch the floor.

- Place your hands on your shoulders and turn the palms upward. Now raise both hands as if you were lifting something over your head. Stretch all the way up. Slowly lower your hands. Do this three times. You will feel tension in the arm muscles. Do this exercise with your head back and then with your head forward.

- Bring one knee up so you are standing on one foot. Pull the knee upward with your hands. Then lower the leg and do the same thing with the other knee. Next, extend each leg as far back as you can, then as far forward. Swing each leg outward and hold it, the longer the better.

If you have trouble with your abdominal muscles, here are two good exercises. The first helps identify the muscles that need added tone; the second, which is more strenuous, will tighten these muscles:

- Draw your stomach muscles in and, at the same time, press your fingertips into the muscles on each side of your abdomen. Apply pressure to these muscles through your fingertips, and then push outward against your fingers. Tighten these muscles, then loosen them and press hard against your fingertips. This exercise helps you both control these muscles and strengthen them.

- The next exercise—sit-ups—may be difficult to do at first, but working at it regularly makes it easier. As always, start slowly and increase the number each day. Lie flat on your back and hook your feet under a bed, couch, or other piece of furniture to stabilize them. Put your hands behind your head and slowly lift your head, bringing your elbows to touch your knees. Then lower yourself back down.

When Is the Best Time to Exercise?

When is the best time to exercise? Morning workouts often are best because they can help you feel ready to face daily stress. A brisk walk or a few movements and stretches get air into your lungs. The downside is that your body may be stiff in the morning and more flexible in the evening. On the other hand, many people find they are too tired to start exercising in the evening.

If you feel like being active in the afternoon or evening, consider rescheduling your other activities. But whatever you do, schedule your exercise as a regular part of your routine. Exercise sessions should be spread out over the week and each exercise activity interlude need not take more than ten or fifteen minutes, although a half-hour is ideal.

If you have heart disease, you should exercise before you eat. Aerobic exercise before a meal can effectively get the blood flowing to your heart and lungs. Diabetics should exercise after they eat, within two hours of the meal. If you wait three or more hours after a meal or exercise in the morning before breakfast, your blood sugar will be too low. Exercise can lower a diabetic person's blood sugar. Have a small snack before exercising and bring a small snack with you if you plan to exercise for over an hour.

By choosing the activities you like, and exercising at a convenient time, you will be more likely to keep exercising regularly and enjoying the many benefits exercise can give your blood pressure.

Stop Exercising if You Experience . . .

Chest pain	Fatigue
Shortness of breath	Heart racing
Dizziness	Joint pain
Nausea	Faintness
Muscle pain	Vertigo
Pain in neck or jaw	

Call your doctor immediately if you experience any of these symptoms.

How Much Exercise Is Best?

For the greatest overall health benefits experts recommend that you do twenty to thirty minutes of exercise or activity three or more times a week. However, if you are unable to do this level of activity, you can still gain substantial health benefits by simply upping your activity levels in your daily life.

ROUTINES FOR THE UNENTHUSIASTIC EXERCISER

If you don't want to exercise daily, but do want to do *some* exercise regularly, set up a three-times-a-week schedule. If you're a city dweller who lives in an apartment house, an easy exercise is to start off walking up one flight of stairs once a day. Then increase it to two times a day. Continue by climbing two flights a day, progressing to two flights twice a day. Then move on to three flights and so on.

Since I live on the third floor, I use the three-flight program. Walking up steps is one of the simplest means of exercise. To date, the best use I've seen of this method has been made by a colleague who walks up twelve flights of stairs every morning.

ROUTINES FOR THE MODERATE EXERCISER

Moderate activities include some of the things you may already be doing during a day or week, such as gardening and housework. These activities can be done in short spurts—ten minutes here, eight minutes there. Alone, each of these activities does not have a great effect on your health, but regularly accumulating thirty minutes of activity over the course of the day can result in substantial heath benefits.

To be more active throughout your day, take advantage of any chance to get up and move around. Here are some examples:

- Take a short walk around the block, up the road, or even to the mailbox.
- Rake leaves, scrub the floor, take out the garbage.
- Play actively with youngsters.
- Walk up and down the stairs; don't take the elevator.
- Take an activity break—get up and stretch or walk briskly.
- Park your car a little farther away; get off the bus before your stop and walk the rest of the way.

Don't allow physical activity to become an unwelcome chore; rather, make the most of the opportunities you have to be active.

ROUTINES FOR THE ATHLETE

Moderate or low-impact exercises such as competitive sports or races as well as running, tennis, handball, soccer, or basketball can provide long-term benefits. More vigorous exercises can be especially helpful when done regularly. They condition the heart and lungs, and lower blood pressure by making you stronger and more flexible—inside and out. So if you like these sorts of activities, incorporate them into your life on a regular basis.

Aerobic Activity

Aerobic activity is an important addition to moderate-intensity exercise. Aerobic exercise is any extended activity that makes you breathe hard while using the large muscle groups at a regular, even pace. Aerobic activities strengthen your heart and lower your blood pressure. Some aerobic activities include:

Brisk walking	Bicycling
Aerobic dancing	Ice or roller skating
Jogging/running	Swimming
Racket sports	Treadmills

Note: Jumping into ice water when you are overheated is not good for people with hypertension. The icy water can contract blood vessels. The same advice goes for jumping into an icy shower after you exercise.

YOUR TARGET ZONE

To get the most health benefits from aerobic activity, you should exercise at a level strenuous enough to raise your heart rate to your target zone. Your target zone is 50 to 75 percent of your maximum heart rate (the fastest your heart can beat). To find your zone, look for the category closest to your age in the chart below and read across the line. For example, if you are thirty-five years old, your target heart rate zone is 93–138 beats per minute.

To see if you are exercising within your target heart rate zone, count the number of pulse beats at your wrist or neck for fifteen seconds, then multiply by four to get the beats per minute. Your heart should be beating within your target heart rate zone. If your heart is beating faster than your target heart rate, you are exercising too hard and should slow down. If your heart is beating slower than your target heart rate, you should exercise a little harder.

Age	Target Heart Rate Zone (50–75%)
20–30 years	95–142 beats per minute
31–40 years	90–135 beats per minute
41–50 years	85–127 beats per minute
51–60 years	80–120 beats per minute
61+ years	75–113 beats per minute

When you begin your exercise program, aim for the lower part of your target zone (50 percent). As you get into better shape, slowly build up to the higher part of your zone (75 percent). If exercising within your target zone seems too hard, exercise at a pace that is comfortable. You will find that with time you can slowly increase your target zone.

> ### *Water or Sports Drinks?*
>
> Water makes 60 to 70 percent of your body weight. It is vital to maintain your body's fluid level. Whether you drink water or a sports drink is a matter of choice. A sports drink contains carbohydrate, often in the form of sugars and electrolytes. Drinks with a high carbohydrate content can delay absorption of water and cause cramps, nausea, or diarrhea and add to your total daily calories.

A Word About Fluids

You can survive a month without food, but only three days without water. When you sweat, you lose water, which must be replaced. Drink fluids before, during, and after workouts.

Keep Going

If you find yourself avoiding exercise, think about why. Do you hate the activity? Try another version of exercise; perhaps another sport. If you're walking, buy a bicycle. If you're dancing, try walking. If the climate prevents you from getting outside, set up a stationary cycle. Or you can alternate your activities, so there is more variety in your exercise program. If you have trouble sticking with your program, finding an exercise buddy may help. Fifty-one men enrolled in a hospital-based exercise program in Peoria, Illinois, were twice as likely to continue their program for a year if their wives or friends exercised with them. Exercises can make you look and feel great. You don't have to build huge muscles or develop a model figure. Muscles and a flat stomach mostly depend on your genes and body shape. But you *can* gain grace, poise, and pleasure. The side effects of exercise are almost all positive.

CHAPTER 30

Walking Your Blood Pressure Down

U nlike tennis, running, skiing, rock climbing, and other activities that have become popular, walking for fitness has withstood the test of time. American historical figures who liked to walk include Emerson and Thoreau. Among American presidents, the most famous walkers included Jefferson, Lincoln, and Truman. Walking is the only exercise in which the rate of participation does not decline in the middle and later years. In a national survey the highest percentage of regular walkers for any group was men 65 years of age and older.

According to the University of Massachusetts Center for Health and Fitness, a brisk forty-minute walk can reduce your blood pressure. Even without weight loss, another study of a group of older women showed that as little as thirty-five minutes of walking three times a week can help lower blood pressure.

Walking, Step by Step

Walking isn't "too easy to do much good," as some think. Studies show that when done briskly on a regular schedule, walking can improve the ability to consume oxygen, lower resting heart rate, reduce blood pressure, and increase the efficiency of the heart, lungs, and blood vessels. It also burns calories—actually about one-third the amount of calories per mile that running does—all while being virtually injury-free. Walking also has several unique advantages:

Working and Walking

Not everyone sits down when they are working. Even in this age of comput-
ers, many jobs still require some walking. Here is a list of occupations and
the estimated number of miles walked daily:

Accountant	1.8	Nurse	5
Architect	2.3	Reporter	2.1
Banker	2	Salesperson, retail	3.5
Dentist	.9	Secretary	2.2
Doctor	2.5	Wait-person	3.3
Editor	1.3		

- Almost everyone can do it.
- You can do it almost any time.
- You can do it alone or in a group.
- You can do it almost anywhere.
- It doesn't cost anything.

In some weight-loss and conditioning studies walking actually has
proven to be more effective than running and other more exciting activities. Walking can also exert a favorable influence on personal habits. Smokers who begin walking often cut down or quit. I believe there are several
reasons for this. It is difficult to exercise vigorously if you are smoking, and
when you are in better physical condition, you also feel you want to improve other aspects of your life. Walking gives you a feeling of getting
someplace, even if you walk in a circular route. Walking is also virtually injury free and has the lowest dropout rate of any form of exercise.

How to Walk

I recommend walking, not meandering or shuffling, or strolling or saun-
tering. When you walk to lower your blood pressure, gain pep, and improve your health, you have to develop an efficient walking style:

- Hold your head up, erect, and keep your back straight and stomach as flat as possible. Your toes should point straight ahead and your arms should swing loosely at your sides.

- Land on the heel of the foot and roll forward to drive off the ball of the foot. Walking only on the ball of the foot, or in a flat-footed style, may cause fatigue and soreness.

- Take long, easy strides, but don't strain for distance. When walking up or down hills, or at a very rapid pace, lean forward slightly.

- Breathe deeply, with your mouth open; it's more comfortable this way.

Note: Researchers at the University of Florida found that people with HBP may be "negatively affected" by using hand weights on their walks. The scientists measured the effects of carrying one- to three-pound weights while using a treadmill. The energy demands on their bodies went up as the weights increased. Hand weights may be beneficial for weight loss and endurance, but it is not for people with high blood pressure.

Clothing You Need

A comfortable pair of shoes is all you need. Actually, any running shoes are good for walking, as are lighter trail and hiking boots and casual shoes with rubber or crepe rubber soles. Whatever kind of shoe you select, it should have good arch support and heels elevated just slightly above the sole. Choose a shoe with material that breathes, such as leather or nylon mesh.

Dress with an eye for the weather. As a general rule you want to wear lighter clothing than the temperature seems to indicate, as walking generates lots of body heat. In cold weather, it is better to wear several layers of light clothing than one or two heavy layers. The extra layers trap heat, and you can shed layers easily if you get warm. A wool cap and scarf will also trap body heat; as much as 20 percent of body heat can be lost from an unprotected neck and head. Wear gloves too; they not only keep your hands warm, they also prevent the loss of body heat.

Even in rainy weather, avoid wearing rubberized or plastic suits, shirts, or pants. If you want to wear some kind of rubberized rain gear, wear an open-weave cotton undershirt or some other shirt that allows air to circulate around your body. In hot weather, if you feel dizzy, weak, light-headed, and/or excessively fatigued, or your sweating stops, stop immediately.

Warm-up and Conditioning Exercises

While walking is good for your legs, heart, and lungs, it is not a complete exercise. People who limit themselves to walking, and do no other exercise, tend to become stiff and inflexible; it also allows the muscles of the back of the legs to become tight. Walking will not improve muscle tone of, nor strengthen, your trunk and upper body. These conditions can lead to poor posture and lower back pain. The following exercises are designed to increase flexibility and serve as a warm-up for walking. About five minutes of warm-up should be enough.

Stretch: Stand facing a wall an arm's length away. Lean forward and place the palms of your hands flat against the wall, slightly below shoulder height. Keep your back straight, heels firmly on the floor, and slowly bend your elbows until your forehead touches the wall. Tuck your hips toward the wall and hold the position for 20 seconds. Repeat the exercise with your knees slightly flexed.

Reach and Bend: Stand erect with your feet shoulder width apart and your arms extended overhead. Reach as high as possible while keeping your heels on the floor and hold for ten counts. Flex your knees slightly and bend slowly at the waist, touching the floor between your feet with your fingers. (If you cannot touch your feet, not to worry; don't strain.) Hold for 10 counts; repeat the entire sequence 2 to 5 times.

Knee-pull: Lie flat on your back with your legs extended and your arms at your sides. Raise your legs, bending your knees. Lock your arms around your legs just below your knees and pull your knees to your chest, raising your buttocks slightly off the floor. Hold for 10 to 15 counts. (If this is difficult, you may find it easier to lock arms behind your knees.) Repeat this exercise 3 to 5 times.

Sit-up: Several versions of the sit-up are listed in reverse order of difficulty (easiest one listed first, most difficult one last). Start with the sit-up that you can do three times without strain. When you are able to do 10 repetitions of a particular sit-up without great difficulty, move on to a more difficult version.

1. Lie flat, then curl your head forward until you can see past your feet. Hold for a second or two; repeat 3 to 10 times.

2. Lie flat on your back with your arms at your sides, your knees slightly bent. Roll forward, lifting your upper body. Repeat exercise 3 to 10 times.

3. Lie flat on your back with your arms at your sides, palms down and knees slightly bent. Roll forward to sitting position. Repeat exercise 3 to 10 times.

4. Lie flat on your back with your arms crossed on your chest and your knees slightly bent. Roll forward to sitting position. Repeat exercise 3 to 10 times.

5. Lie flat on your back with your hands laced in back of your head and your knees slightly bent. Roll forward to the sitting position. Repeat exercise 3 to 5 times.

Cool Down After Your Walk

After a brisk walk, or any aerobic exercise, slow down gradually. A few minutes of a leisurely stroll will allow your body to cool down gradually. Abrupt stopping, just like abrupt starting of exertion, can cause dizziness. A few stretches after your walk will loosen you up and ease you back into your normal routine.

Other Options for Moderate Sports

Walking, no matter how convenient, may not fit your schedule. Here are some other choices:

Run in place: One simple exercise that requires no equipment is running in place. You can start by running for two minutes and increase the time, as long as it feels comfortable.

Bicycling: Outdoor cycling is an excellent and always popular form of exercise. Some of the new bicycles are light in weight, so that riding is comfortable and pleasant. In many areas, cycle clubs have one-day or even longer trips. You may find the group activity a help in getting committed to your exercise regimen.

Exercise bicycle: The moderate daily exerciser might consider an exercise bicycle for home use. There are many models from which to choose, and I've seen one at every garage sale I've been to for the past few years.

Sports and High Blood Pressure

A large study compared the health of men who were involved in sports, and those who were not. Of the men who had never participated in any kind of exercise or sports, 13.9 percent had high blood pressure, as opposed to a rate of 8.2 percent of those who engaged in some type of sports.

Select one that has a device for controlling the degree of resistance against which you must pedal. Start with a low degree of resistance and slowly increase it as you progressively increase the amount of time you spend pedaling.

Swimming: Swimming is excellent exercise. Water provides the same kind of resistance that the exercise bicycle does. To increase the amount of exercise, simply increase the number of laps you swim if you are using a pool, and then increase the speed at which you do the distance.

Running or Jogging: Jogging has become very popular in recent years. However, it should be done with an element of caution. Carried past a certain point, jogging can lead to foot and knee problems.

Cross-country skiing: This sport requires far less technical skill than downhill skiing, and you can move along as fast or as slowly as you wish. A plus is that the skis are less expensive than the downhill equipment. All you need is an open field or city park and some snow.

For more information on sports and exercise write: The President's Council on Physical Fitness and Sports, 701 Pennsylvania Avenue, NW, Suite 250, Washington, DC 20004 (202) 272-3421.

Exercise/Sports Clubs

If you like exercise and recognize the benefits, consider joining a health club. I have spoken with many people who say that the club helped them get on an exercise/sports program and stay on it. One patient told me that she is committed to exercise/sports because she paid for the club membership and feels it's a waste if she does not attend. Before you join any club or group, make sure the facilities are clean and there is a qualified instructor to help you perform your exercises/sports, and to help you avoid injury.

Keep Going

Set your sights on short-term as well as long-term goals. For example, your long-term goal is to lose weight and lower your systolic and diastolic pressure. Your short-term goals are to walk every day for fifteen minutes, and then to walk one mile, and so on. Gradually you will meet both your short-term and long-term goals.

PART IV

Hypertension Drugs

Drugs are powerful chemicals. Along with their benefits, they also have potential for harm. You need to know what antihypertensive drugs are and how they work.

New drugs, newly popular herbal cures, and new ways of delivering the drugs are being introduced every day. Here is an overview of many of these medications—and some caveats on their use.

CHAPTER 31

About Antihypertensive Drugs

Just fifty years ago a diagnosis of hypertension was a death sentence. Even then, we knew that high blood pressure could progress to a stroke or heart attack, but in those days, when I first started my practice as a physician, we had little help to offer our patients. The only treatment to reduce the blood pressure consisted of a low-salt diet, bed rest, and possibly the use of "sleeping pills." The rice diet (see Chapter 11) helped some people but was not suitable for many hypertensives. With the introduction of antihypertensive drugs this gloomy picture changed.

Nondrug Therapy

Drug treatment of long-term high blood pressure can significantly reduce the death rate from heart disease and stroke. However, the use of these medicines is not always the best choice. People with mild hypertension and no heart problems usually can bring blood pressure down to normal levels in about a year after starting lifestyle changes. These changes can also help the patient manage HBP over the long term, since hypertension does not go away. This makes medications unnecessary.

Whenever possible, nondrug therapies such as alcohol and sodium restriction, weight reduction, elimination of smoking, relaxation techniques, exercise, and stress control should be used to lower the blood pressure before turning to the more risky use of medications.

Alas, nondrug therapy is not always enough. For people with diabetes, controlling both blood pressure and blood glucose levels is imperative for preventing serious complications. Let me stress again: You must work with your doctor to find the right treatment for you. If drugless methods do not lower your pressure enough, you still have many choices.

Combined Treatment

A single-drug regimen can often control mild to moderate hypertension. More severe hypertension often requires a combination of two or more drugs. A blend of drugless methods with appropriate medications is often the best approach to hypertension. Since the value of medication for many people is obvious, I would in no way suggest that one should avoid medication or stop taking it if it has been prescribed by your doctor. (Never stop taking your medicine suddenly or without your doctor's knowledge.) Patients should incorporate nondrug therapies along with medication to obtain the best results.

Just How Valuable Is Medication?

The positive results obtained with drugs have been demonstrated in many research projects and studies. The results of three of those studies, which were done more than a decade ago, are described below. (Note: Under today's medical ethics, we do not allow any patients to go untreated for research purposes. Technology has advanced enough to make many human studies unnecessary, and soon, animal studies will also be a thing of the past.)

- A group of seventy men who had diastolic blood pressure readings ranging from 115 to129 mm Hg were left untreated. Of this group, four died of cardiovascular disease and twenty-three had serious complications from hypertension.

- A group of seventy-three men with the same diastolic pressure readings were treated with medication; none died of cardiovascular disease, and only two had serious complications.

- In a study of men with diastolic blood pressure readings ranging from 90 to 114 mm Hg, nineteen who were untreated died of cardiovascular disease; fifty-seven had complications. In the treated group only eight died of cardiovascular disease and fourteen had complications.

Should You Start Drug Treatment?

Although medications can be both life-saving and health-preserving, there is controversy over which medications should be used and when they should be started. Before we consider the problems of when to treat and how, let's review accepted treatments. Anyone with elevated blood pressure, no matter how mild, should be monitored. Blood pressure should be checked regularly and, depending upon the degree of elevation, various tests may help to evaluate what programs would be best to encourage total health. How often blood pressure should be checked is a function of many factors. However, most experts believe a good rule of thumb is that the higher the readings, the more frequent the monitoring.

Most physicians agree that drug treatment is indicated when the patient's diastolic blood pressure exceeds 100 mm Hg because complications may occur at that level. For those patients whose pressure is below 100 mm Hg diastolic but over 80 mm Hg diastolic, several questions should be asked. Do they need drug treatment? If so, how much? What kind? When should it be started? These are important questions, and are often made by the patient and the doctor reviewing the options and working together.

High Blood Pressure and Complications from Other Diseases

Some complications may develop from other diseases.

Gout can injure the blood vessels as well as the kidneys and the joints of the body; immediate treatment is essential. Complications may result in the loss of kidney function so that the kidneys are unable to clear the body of the waste products of metabolism.

Heart damage is equally serious. Changes in electrocardiogram readings may indicate the heart is having difficulty pumping against increased pressure in the vascular system. As the need for more blood develops, the heart muscles will enlarge and thicken, causing heart failure.

Eye complications that can occur include a leakage of blood from very tiny blood vessels into the back of the eye. The physician can directly examine the back of the eye with an ophthalmoscope. This instrument allows the physician to see this leakage and any spasms of the blood vessels. The presence of other conditions heightens the need to treat hypertension.

Risk Factor Complications

Treatment with drugs is often indicated for people with the following complicating risk factors:

High blood cholesterol: People with high blood cholesterol levels face a greater risk of heart disease than do others. The relationship is very direct: The risk rises as the blood cholesterol level goes up. A total cholesterol level of less than 200 mg dl is thought to be desirable.

Smoking: People who smoke face a higher risk of coronary disease than those who do not, because smoking directly increases both systolic and diastolic blood pressure.

Diabetes: Diabetes constitutes an increased risk both directly, as a disease that damages blood vessels and thereby increases the dangers of various types of cardiovascular disease, and indirectly, as a disease that requires careful medical monitoring.

Heredity: A family history of complications due to hypertension is extremely significant. The presence of these complications within a family indicates a genetic influence, and the statistics bear this out. Because of an inherent predisposition, the complications of hypertension often occur in such people at lower levels of pressure than is the case with others.

Obesity: Weighing more than you should is a major risk factor in the advent of HBP, which then can lead to strokes, cardiovascular disease, heart disease, kidney disease, and eye disease. High blood pressure in conjunction with any of these diseases indicates that blood pressure control is both essential and urgent.

Age: Blood pressure must be measured in older persons with special care, because they often suffer from vascular stiffness. Many older people respond well to lifestyle modifications.

Pregnancy: It is important for women to follow the directions of their doctor.

Initiating Drug Therapy

Once it is decided that drug treatment is needed, what should be done? First, it is important that anyone with HBP continue to use standard non-drug treatments: weight control, exercise, salt reduction, a diet low in cholesterol (with adequate nutritional intake), reduction of alcohol intake, elimination of smoking, stress control, and rest. When medicines are prescribed, careful monitoring is essential to determine the correct dosage and to spot any adverse reactions or side effects. For the best results, you must be willing and able to work with your physician to monitor your drug use. Adhering to the program and cooperating with your doctor in the medical follow-up is vital.

Medications to Lower Blood Pressure

Here are the general classifications of the drugs most often used to lower high blood pressure and how each type works. Many wonderful prescription medicines are available at this time. But because pharmacology is moving so rapidly, new medicines are constantly being introduced. Every day we read about new medications, better delivery systems, and even new uses for drugs that have been used for years.

Most people with mild HBP can control their blood pressure with non-drug lifestyle modifications and one drug. However, if the drug that your doctor prescribes isn't effective, or the side effects are intolerable, report this as soon as possible. Your doctor may change the dosage of your medication or prescribe another drug. By using a combination of two or more

---

Medication Mood Swings

Some antihypertensive medications may cause depression or other changes in mood. One group known to do this is the beta-blockers. Such mood changes are rare, but if they do occur they may be severe. A wide range of medications is available for the treatment of high blood pressure, and small changes in the medication formula may be all that is needed. Discuss your reactions to any prescription with your doctor.

drugs, doctors can probably provide you with a medication that lowers your blood pressure and has no or minimal side effects.

When using combination therapy, your doctor often looks for medications that enhance each other's effectiveness and also reduce each other's side effects. A combination of drugs can also be tailored to take into account, and even ameliorate, any other medical problems you may have.

DIURETICS

For several decades diuretics have been used for lowering high blood pressure. They sometimes are called "water pills" because they flush excess sodium and water from the body in the urine. This lessens the amount of fluid in the blood. Sodium is also flushed out of the blood vessel walls, allowing the blood vessels to dilate. As a result, there is less pressure on the blood vessels. Diuretics come in different brands and doctors prescribe different kinds for different people.

Diuretics can have unpleasant side effects; the most common are:

gastrointestinal disturbances	reduced potassium
muscle cramps	photosensitivity
impotence	weakness
increased urination	rashes
increased blood sugar	

Short-term side effects of diuretics may also include increases of cholesterol and glucose levels and biochemical changes that affect the levels of magnesium and calcium in the body. There may also be an increase in uric acid, triggering gout.

If you use a diuretic, your doctor should carefully monitor its effects to be sure that your level of potassium, which passes out of your body with urine, is sufficient. The dosage must be increased or decreased, depending on your response. Signs of potassium insufficiency are weakness, leg cramps, and a feeling of chronic fatigue. If potassium loss is severe, it will interfere with the normal contractions of the heart. To prevent this, blood tests should be run to determine the potassium levels, and correct action should be taken if necessary. In some cases the changes connected with severe potassium loss will appear on an electrocardiogram.

A loss of potassium can be overcome by increasing potassium in your diet. Bananas and dried fruits are high in potassium. You can also drink orange juice, which is high in potassium. Supplements, in the form of potassium pills or a liquid, can be given to counteract the problem of potassium loss. Controlling potassium loss can also be done by using a drug formula that will help retain potassium.

How successful are diuretics in treating hypertension? Many studies indicate that 80 percent of patients with high blood pressure can be treated successfully with these drugs. It is the simplest medication and causes the least imbalance in the body's physiology, and it has the fewest side effects. Diuretics have reduced the incidence of stroke by a significant degree and have also lowered the risk for hypertensive-related heart attacks.

There are three types of diuretics: thiazides, loop diuretics, and potassium-sparing agents. Thiazides often are the basis for high blood pressure treatment. They can be taken alone for mild hypertension or used in combination with other types of drugs. For patients for whom simple thiazide medication does not control blood pressure, what's known as step therapy must be tried. In this type of therapy, strong and stronger medicines are added progressively until the proper control is obtained. Increasing the drug potency strengthens its antihypertensive effect, producing changes in all levels of body function. Step therapy can take different forms, involving different combinations of drugs.

Many authorities now feel that one need no longer start with the thiazide diuretics, as was done in the past, but other drugs can be used instead. At present, progressive step therapy is the most widely used treatment and historically the most successful.

BETA-BLOCKERS

Medications that reduce the number of nerve impulses that occur in the heart and blood vessels and also slow certain metabolic processes are called beta-blockers. This reduction slows the heart, which beats less often and with less contracting force—so blood pressure drops and the heart doesn't work as hard as it normally does. Beta-blocker patients seem to have a lowered risk for a second heart attack or sudden death after a first heat attack. (Note: This lowered heart attack rate may not be true for an older patient.)

These drugs are not as effective as ACE inhibitors (explained below) in people with, or at risk for, kidney disease. Beta-blockers can narrow bronchial airways and constrict blood vessels in people with asthma or Raynaud's disease; digestive problems and sexual problems are part of the side effects. Some beta-blockers tend to lower HDL (good guys); this effect is most noted in smokers.

Fatigue, depression, memory loss, and lethargy are among some of the other possible side effects. There may also be sleep disturbances: Some people report vivid dreams and nightmares, depression, and memory loss. Drinking alcohol while on beta-blockers can sometimes increase the chance of side effects such as dizziness or tiredness. It is dangerous to discontinue treatment suddenly; your doctor should be involved with a gradual withdrawal.

ANGIOTENSIN CONVERTING ENZYME (ACE) INHIBITORS

ACE inhibitors are becoming increasingly popular. They block a kidney-produced hormone that narrows blood vessels, causing blood pressure to rise. This type of medication has successfully battled all types of hypertension.

ACE inhibitors are recommended as first-line treatment for people with diabetes and kidney damage, for some heart attack survivors, and for patients with heart failure when they are also taking diuretics. A recent study offers sound medical proof that, like beta-blockers and aspirin, ACE inhibitors can improve a patient's odds of surviving a heart attack. These drugs are expensive, but one study showed that ACE inhibitors decreased the risk of death and reduced hospital visits, saving over $1,500 per patient over a three-year period.

Side effects are uncommon but may include a rash, cough, headache, a severe drop in blood pressure, and allergic reactions. A recent study found that although ACE inhibitors can protect against kidney disease, they also cause the kidney to retain potassium, which can result in heart problems if levels become too high. Because of this, they are not generally given with potassium-sparing diuretics or potassium supplements. Another recent study showed that ACE inhibitors slow the progress of nondiabetic kidney disease.

CALCIUM CHANNEL BLOCKERS

Approximately six million people take calcium channel blockers to treat hypertension. These drugs block entry of calcium into blood vessel walls and the muscle cells of the heart, relaxing and dilating vessels. There are two kinds—short-acting, which produce rapid relaxation, and long-

> ## Broadening the Use of ACE Inhibitors
>
> In November of 1999, there was an exciting news story on TV and in the newspapers: The drug ramipril, an ACE inhibitor, which has been marketed for more than eight years to combat high blood pressure, has turned out to substantially lower the risk of heart attack, stroke, bypass surgery, and diabetes and its complications in those who have heart disease. It is not immediately clear whether the findings about ramipril will hold for the other ACE inhibitors on the market.

acting, which work gradually for a longer period. The long-acting drugs are the newest and most commonly used.

Calcium channel blockers have an immediate effect on reducing blood pressure, but they have been linked to some problems, and some results are poor compared to those of other medicines. Grapefruit juice appears to boost the effect of these drugs when taken by some elderly people. No one should take these drugs or stop taking them without understanding their use and discussing the medication with their doctor.

Of major concern are reports of an increased risk of death and serious heart events from abrupt drops in blood pressure in people taking the short-acting forms. Another study reported that women who took channel blockers had a higher risk for heart attack than those on diuretics. This study, however, may not reflect the current trend toward taking long-acting calcium channel blockers.

Side effects may include swelling of legs, dizziness, gum disease, palpitation, headache, flushing, and constipation. Some of these negative side effects of calcium channel blockers may be reduced when they are taken with beta-blockers.

ALPHA-BLOCKERS

These medications work on the body's nervous system. They lower pressure by blocking the impulse to tighten the muscles in the walls of your smaller arteries. Alpha-blockers also reduce the effects of some hormones (noradrenaline and adrenaline) that narrow blood vessels. An additional benefit of alpha-blockers is that they lower blood cholesterol and triglyceride levels; for people at risk for a heart attack, alpha-blockers offer a double benefit. For older men with prostate problems, alpha-blockers improve urine flow, so they reduce nighttime visits to the bathroom. Alpha-blockers, which are both short- and long-term acting, are also good for young people who may not be candidates for beta-blockers.

Side effects can include dizziness or feelings of faintness, nausea, and a pounding heartbeat. Alpha-blockers slow your body's time to respond to natural changes in blood pressure.

ALPHA-BETA-BLOCKERS

These drugs work in the same way alpha-blockers do, but also slow the heartbeat so less blood is pumped through the blood vessels.

NERVOUS SYSTEM INHIBITORS

Many blood pressure medications work to relax blood vessels to allow more blood flow. They prevent your brain from sending signals to your nervous system to speed up your heart rate and to narrow your blood vessels. Also called central adrenergic inhibitors, these aren't used as often as they once were because of the side effects. Your doctor may recommend a central-acting agent if you're prone to panic attacks, you have low blood sugar, or you're going through drug or alcohol withdrawal. These drugs can help reduce the symptoms of these conditions.

Side effects include fatigue and a zombielike feeling that some patients find intolerable. It is also very dangerous to stop these agents suddenly; your blood pressure can rebound very high in a very short time. Discuss with your physician any changes you may be contemplating.

VASODILATORS

Just as the name says, these drugs dilate the arteries. They are usually combined with other drugs, especially diuretics and beta-blockers. The side effects include growth of hair and some vitamin deficiencies. (Testing these drugs resulted in the development of minoxidil, a drug that when applied to a balding scalp can grow hair in some people.)

In the Test Tubes

Medical researchers are at work developing new drugs and working on new strategies to make people with HBP more comfortable and to keep pressure low enough to avoid damage to other body systems. They are investi-

Medication Alerts

Before taking any medicine, your doctor should be told if:

- You have ever had an allergic reaction to any medicine.

- You are pregnant or plan to become pregnant.

- You have had any medical problems other than hypertension.

Be sure you know what you are taking:

- Take any medicine exactly as directed, at the right time.

- To avoid mistakes, do not take medicine in the dark; always check labels.

- Never mix medicines in one container.

- Store medicines away from heat and direct sunlight, and away from moisture.

- Do not keep outdated medicine.

Precautions while using medicine:

- Never lend or give your medicine to anyone else.

- If you have any adverse reactions, call your doctor.

- Carry a day's supply or more of your medicine with you, especially when you travel.

- Keep a list of all your prescriptions in your wallet or someplace where it can be found.

- Understand why you are taking a medication, and how it works in your body.

gating ways to keep arteries open and wide to ease blood flow. They are also working to ensure that certain compounds that fight high blood pressure remain in your body for longer periods. Methods to stop the narrowing of blood vessels and the retention of sodium are other subjects that are now being researched.

There is a connection between people who develop essential hypertension and their genetic makeup. But it is not easy to find the precise link, since HBP is multifaceted and seems to involve the interaction of many genes. Great progress has recently been made in mapping the human genes. Many specific genes linked to a specific disease have been spotted; perhaps as a result of this sort of genetic research high blood pressure will soon become a problem of the past.

The Best Way to Take Your Medicine

Ideally, a drug should enter the body slowly and steadily, go directly to the problem site while bypassing healthy systems and tissues, do its job, and then disappear. Unfortunately, the typical methods for delivery of drugs—pills and injections—rarely achieve this goal.

Drugs that are swallowed may not be able to cross the intestinal membrane and enter the bloodstream. Also, some therapeutic proteins and enzymes can actually be digested. If a drug does enter the blood, it is hard to judge how much of the drug is needed to reach its therapeutic level. Injections are also often unsatisfactory because they are expensive and difficult to administer.

New ideas in the delivery of medications are ingenious: The now-familiar drug-impregnated skin patches, for instance, bypass the digestive system altogether and have worked well with many hypertension medications, providing a slow, steady drug delivery directly to the bloodstream. However, only very small drug molecules can get into the body through the skin.

A nasal delivery system for insulin (used to treat diabetes) has been developed and may soon be in general use. Nasal delivery systems are now being investigated for a number of medications. Bio-erodible implants are being developed as well as thin waferlike implants. Another drug delivery vehicle that has been viewed as promising is a microscopic bubble of fatty molecules that surrounds the drug and carries it through most of the digestive system.

Very promising are prolonged-release drugs; these can provide more medication during early morning hours, when patients are at highest risk of heart attack or stroke.

All of the advances in drug development and delivery are the result of ingenious ideas and long years of study and testing. We've come far in the past half-century, and most likely will see many more methods of taking medications.

Ask Your Doctor

If your doctor prescribes a drug to treat your high blood pressure, be sure to ask:

- When it should be taken.

- What you can eat and drink with it, or how long you must wait before and after a meal to take it.

- What other drugs can or cannot be taken at the same time.

- What to do if you run out of a drug.

- What to do if you forget to take a dose.

- If there are any special instructions.

- If the pills can be bought in high dosages and then split with a sharp knife. Note: This doesn't work for capsules or coated pills.

You should also:

- Comparison-shop among pharmacies. Don't stockpile too many medications. Three months' supply is generally sufficient to earn any discount for bulk orders.

- Before any surgery or dental work, tell the physician or dentist that you are taking antihypertensive medications.

High Blood Pressure Drug Overview

Dozens of antihypertensive drugs are available. The most used medications are diuretics, which cause the body to excrete water and salt; ACE inhibitors, which reduce the production of a chemical that causes arteries to constrict; beta-blockers, which ease the heart's pumping action and widen blood vessels; vasodilators, which expand blood vessels; and calcium channel blockers, which help decrease the contractions of the heart and widen blood vessels.

Doctors often recommend beta-blockers or diuretics, which are inexpensive, fairly safe, and effective. Other drugs or combinations are usually recommended for specific problems or to address problems that may arise when a patient has more than one disease. ACE inhibitors should be used as a first-line treatment for people with diabetes and kidney damage. Heart attack survivors are usually given beta-blockers and sometimes ACE inhibitors to prevent a second attack. People with heart failure are often given ACE inhibitors and diuretics; specific drugs in these classes may be particularly beneficial for patients because they reduce enlargement of chambers of the heart. One study showed that diuretics are effective for preventing heart failure after a heart attack.

Because they have a high risk for salt sensitivity, African-Americans are usually prescribed diuretics. Isolated high systolic pressure is treated with diuretics; one study found that when a beta-blocker was added to a diuretic, the risk of heart failure was cut in half. Some experts warn against taking short-acting calcium channel blockers, which may increase the risk of heart problems and even death. Some studies are also suggesting that calcium channel blockers may increase the risk for certain cancers, including breast cancer, and also for bleeding during surgery.

Handling Drug Side Effects

If you are taking drugs you should immediately notify your physician if any complications occur. However, you must weigh the possible dangers of the medicine against the dangers of high blood pressure, and the choice must be made on the basis of a comparative evaluation of each. In the end, the complications of seriously elevated blood pressure are invariably more severe and life-threatening than are the side effects of medication. For that reason, treatment is generally indicated despite the possible side effects. To complete the picture of drug therapy for hypertension, one must acknowledge a vast array of medications under development, offering the potential for better control of hypertension with less danger.

While you are taking any antihypertensive drugs, avoid alcohol, other medications taken without a doctor's permission, strenuous exercise, hot rooms, or a diet too low in salt (unless your doctor has advised it). The new antihypertensive drugs are extremely powerful, and while they can do an outstanding job in reducing many of the complications of hypertension, they also have the potential for causing serious side effects. You must be under the careful monitoring of a physician when you take any prescription medications.

What should you do if you are taking one of these medicines and find yourself suddenly feeling weak, faint, and possibly nauseated to the point of vomiting? Lie down at once with your feet at a level higher than your head. This will help return the blood to your head; the decrease in pressure caused the blood to leave your head. Unless the loss of pressure is extreme, assuming this position should relieve the reaction. If it does not, you will need emergency medical care, including medications, to return your pressure to a better level.

To avoid this situation in the first place, do not get up suddenly or rapidly when you begin to take any of these medications. Give yourself a chance to determine how your body reacts to the reduction in pressure. In elderly people, this drop in pressure can be serious, causing complications to the kidneys as well as brain damage.

Physicians have also been concerned about the long-term effects of antihypertensive drugs on mental processes. A recent study found that brain scans of people who took calcium channel blockers or a class of diuretics detected changes in brain tissue; those who took beta-blockers had no such changes. In spite of these worrisome reports and expert recommendations of other drugs for first-line treatment, the number of calcium channel blocker prescriptions has increased and the number of prescriptions for beta-blockers has decreased in recent years. If you find yourself experiencing unpleasant mental or emotional changes, consult your physician. Another medication may be more appropriate for you.

A Word About Over-the-Counter Medications

Although mild and relatively uncommon, interactions involving over-the-counter drugs can produce unwanted results or make HBP medications less effective. It's especially important to know about drug interactions if you are taking prescribed standard medicines and over-the-counter drugs at the same time. A list of some of the OTC medications that have a high salt content is on page 74.

Some drugs can also interact with foods and beverages, as well as with health conditions such as diabetes, kidney disease, and high blood pressure. Here are a few drug interaction cautions for some common OTC ingredients:

- Avoid alcohol if you are taking any antihypertensive drug.
- Avoid OTC drugs with a high sodium content if you take any diuretic: Check the labels.

- Do not take drugs that treat sleeplessness unless you check with your doctor.
- Do not use a laxative when you have stomach pain, nausea, or vomiting.
- Do not take cough/cold or weight control medicines without checking with your doctor if you have hypertension, heart or thyroid disease, diabetes, or prostate problems.
- Many OTC medications sold as decongestants and cold and asthma remedies contain an agent that can raise blood pressure. Read the labels or consult with your pharmacist or physician.

Medications are powerful enough to affect your body, so it is important to read the label and any written warnings that are packaged with any over-the-counter medication. You can never be too cautious when taking medications, especially when in combination. As always, when in doubt consult your physician.

CHAPTER 32

Herbs, Vitamins, and Minerals and Hypertension

Just down the street, between a Chinese restaurant and a pizza parlor, I've noticed a new store: It sells vitamins and minerals in varying doses as well as herbal medicines such as ground roots and leaves. My neighborhood is typical: grocery stores, supermarkets, drugstores, and department stores now often have sections devoted to herbal and supplemental therapies, and stores, such as the one on my street, selling herbal remedies have seemingly sprouted everywhere. Herbal supplements designed as therapy for illnesses are also sold through mail order, TV programs, and the Internet. According to the Food and Drug Administration dietary supplements accounted for $3.3 billion of sales in 1990 and more than $8 billion in sales in 1999. Continued growth is predicted.

Patients as well as the doctors who prescribe them still ask questions about herbs and dietary supplements. In setting up the Dietary Supplement Health and Education Act in 1994 the National Institutes of Health attempted to get some answers. Since hypertension has so few symptoms, and because it is a lifelong health problem, people with hypertension might be vulnerable to some of the aggressive marketing tactics that are often used. There is much misinformation about these products.

Once a dietary supplement is marketed, the Food and Drug Administration has the responsibility for showing that the dietary supplement is unsafe before it can take action to restrict the product's use. For example, this was the case in June of 1997, when the FDA proposed limiting the amount of ephedrine alkaloids in ephedra. The FDA also provided warn-

---

Rauwolfia

The World Health Organization estimates that 4 billion people, 80 percent of the world population, presently use herbal medicine for some aspects of primary health care. Herbal medicine is a component in Western medicine and a common element in Asian medicine and many folk medicines. The Java devil pepper *(Rauwolfia serpentina)* has been used by Hindus since ancient times to treat high blood pressure. There is no information on the safety or the effectiveness of this, or many other, herbals.

---

ings about its hazards, ranging from nervousness, dizziness, and changes in heart rate and blood pressure.

Claims and Quality

Patients should check with their doctor before they take any herbal supplements. I am particularly wary of any product with the following claims or language:

- Secret products.
- Pseudomedical jargon, such as "detoxify," "energize," and "purify."
- Very broad claims, such as a product can cure anything from hypertension to brittle nails.
- Vague "scientific studies" that are not verified.
- Claims that the product has no side effects; most medications that are powerful enough to work have some side effects.
- Accusations that the medical profession, drug companies, and the government suppress information about a particular treatment.

Poor manufacturing practices are not unique to herbal and other dietary supplements. But because there is now such a large market for herbal supplements and therapeutic-strength vitamins and minerals, and, because they are developed and marketed with fewer restrictions than standard medicine, there is the potential for abuse. To help you protect yourself:

- Look for ingredients in products with the U.S.P. notation, which indicates the manufacturer followed standards established by the United

Supplements Associated with Adverse
HBP Reactions

HERB	POSSIBLE HEALTH HAZARD
Coffee and Tea	Caffeine can constrict blood vessels
Comfrey	Obstruction of blood flow to the liver
Ephedra	Can cause high blood pressure, irregular heartbeat
Licorice	Causes body to retain fluids
Lobelia	Can cause rapid heartbeat, low blood pressure
Mistletoe	Increases blood pressure
Rosemary	Increases blood pressure

States Pharmacopeia, a national listing of recognized products. A good source of information about herbals is the Herb Research Foundation, 1007 Pearl Street, Suite 200, Boulder, CO 80302. E-mail: info@herbs.org and homepage: www.herbs.org

- Read the fine print.
- Remember the term "natural" doesn't mean safe.
- Look for nationally known food and drug manufacturers.
- Freshness counts; fresh herbs are generally more potent.
- Don't hesitate to write the company that produces the supplement to ask for more information about the product and any possible side effects. A reputable supplier will be glad to send you information.

Some Supplements Have Promise

Many herbals have a diuretic action that has long been noted and is part of folk medicine. Just like diuretic drugs, they increase blood flow in your kidneys and increase urination. These herbs may be useful in helping prevent bladder infections and kidney problems.

asparagus	linden blossom
fennel	borage

hibiscus	parsley
juniper	sarsaparilla
dandelion	saw palmetto
hawthorn	yarrow

There are also other herbal supplements that you may want to investigate.

Depression: hawthorn, linden blossom, St. John's wort, cramp bark

Stress: cramp bark, hawthorn, linden blossom, yarrow, Siberian ginseng, valerian

Headache: hawthorn, linden blossom, valerian

Aromatherapy has recently become popular. It offers oils to use in relaxing massages and candles for a scented atmosphere. Relaxing fragrances in oils or other products include chamomile, rose, bergamot, and lavender. The massage and stress-lowering self-awareness may be just as important as the fragrances.

High Blood Pressure and Vitamins, Minerals, and Nutrients

Many nutrients are now being tested to find out if they can reduce or eliminate the need for antihypertensive drugs. Unlike drugs, which act almost immediately, vitamins and nutrients take time to work, if they work at all. If you add any nutrients to your diet, allow about three months to see any results. When you change your diet, you should check with your doctor; he or she may want to monitor your blood pressure and determine if lowering the dosage of any standard medicine you take is advisable. Here's some information on the most common herbal supplements thought to be of value in patients with high blood pressure:

Magnesium: High blood pressure can indicate a deficiency in minerals that keep blood pressure in balance. A diet rich in magnesium (see Chapter 18) or magnesium supplements can be helpful. About 80 percent of Americans are thought to be magnesium-deficient, and even if magnesium fails to lower your blood pressure, it can reduce your risk of arterial disease and stroke. Although magnesium is usually safe, an adverse side effect can be diarrhea when too much is taken.

Potassium: A potassium deficiency can cause high blood pressure in some people, so those with high blood pressure should consider taking potassium supplements. Unlike magnesium, too much potassium can be very dangerous (see Chapter 18). A blood test can tell you if you need more potassium. If you are in doubt, eat a banana—a fruit high in potassium.

Fish oils: Recently many studies of fish oils, which contain omega-3 fatty acids, found that fish oil can lower blood pressure, but only modestly, and then only with some people. There are some cardiovascular benefits associated with fish oils. You can take codliver oil supplements, but you must be wary because it is also very high in vitamins A, D, and E. A tuna fish salad from albacore tuna (canned tuna is fine, if you rinse out all the salt) is high in omega-3 fat.

Garlic: Folklore about the abilities of garlic to keep you safe from harm may have some scientific basis. A study in the *British Journal of Clinical Practice* reported that garlic supplements have been able to bring about a significant reduction in blood pressure in patients with mild hypertension. Some researchers claim that garlic raises HDL (good cholesterol) and works against heart disease by dilating the blood vessels, lowering blood pressure, and making the blood less likely to clot. (Besides, it is wonderful in many dishes.) Garlic extract can be bought in health food stores. The amount recommended to lower blood pressure is between 1,500 to 6,000 milligrams a day. Some studies have indicated that garlic can thin the blood—so consult your physician.

Vitamin C: Among other blood-pressure-lowering nutrients is vitamin C in high dosages. Some studies have reported that when high-blood-pressure patients whose pressure was more than 140/90 mm Hg were given 500 milligrams a day of vitamin C, their blood pressure was reduced an average of 9 percent. The benefits began about a month after the vitamin was added to their diets. These dosages can interact harmfully with any medications you are taking. Vitamin C is also a major antioxidant nutrient. It prevents the conversion of nitrates (tobacco smoke and bacon) into cancer-causing substances. Deficiency can lead to slow-healing wounds, nosebleeds, and capillary weakness. Excessive amounts of vitamin C may cause kidney stones.

Multinutritional supplements: Supplements that include vitamin B complex, zinc, vitamin A, and vitamin E have all been thought to help lower blood pressure and reduce the effects of hypertension. They are the subject of several studies.

Other supplements: Coenzyme Q10 is thought to lower blood pressure when amounts of 200 to 300 milligrams are taken daily. Gingko biloba may be dangerous because it may thin the blood.

Fiber: Raw fruits and vegetables, whole grain cereals, oat bran, and seeds are good sources of fiber, which can help with high blood pressure. Drink water often—before you actually feel thirsty; it helps the fiber do its job.

Where to Learn More

Every day we learn more about how foods, herbs, nutrients, and lifestyle interact to help the body keep strong and the vascular system flexible. You can learn more for yourself by writing or calling:

American Herbalist Guild, P.O. Box 1683, Soquel, CA 95073 (408) 464-2441, www.healthworld.com

American Holistic Medical Association, 6728 Old McLean Village Drive, McLean, VA 22101-3906 (703) 556-9728, www.holisticmedicine.org

For problems with any supplement used, call a doctor. He or she in turn can report it to FDA MedWatch by calling (800) FDA-1088 or by going to www.fda.gov/medwatch/report/hcp.htm on the MedWatch Web site.

Much remains unknown about many herbs and dietary supplements, their health benefits and potential risks. However, the availability of a wide range of such products makes it vital for all of us to learn as much as we can. Consumers who decide to take advantage of the expanding market should do so with caution, making sure they have the necessary information and consulting with their doctors.

A Final Word

In writing this book, I have offered alternatives to drug medications for treating hypertension. You may be able to avoid the use of drugs or can use a lower dosage, with nondrug therapies. The nondrug methods will lessen your dependency on medications and your need to deal with their side effects. It is important to remember that you can play a part in controlling hypertension: your diet and your lifestyle can help contribute to successful treatment.

PART V

Shopping and Cooking with High Blood Pressure

Most people are busy these days. They have less time than they used to for shopping, for planning what to eat, and for cooking. Research in the last few years has shown that the way people eat has a lot to do with how healthy they are—and how healthy they stay.

The recipes included in this section will start you cooking with very little salt and little saturated fat—but with lots of flavor. I hope these recipes encourage you to develop and collect your own low-salt and low-fat recipes.

CHAPTER 33

A Life of Healthy Eating: Recipes to Lower Your Blood Pressure

D iet affects the development of high blood pressure. Recently, a study found that one particular eating plan can lower elevated blood pressure. On pages 317–24, I've included the DASH diet, which was developed by the National Institutes of Health just for people with hypertension. This diet has been used by many, and most people find it easy to follow and convenient; best of all it includes many popular food choices.

This section offers you recipes to help you stay on the DASH plan. The recipes have been developed to be low in salt, fat, and saturated fats. Also included are some suggestions to guide you in shopping for food and in choosing portion size. While the DASH eating plan and these recipes are designed for people with elevated blood pressure, they are also heart-healthy meals that you can share with your family.

Low-Salt/Low-Fat Recipes

Here are twenty-five recipes, as well as an all-purpose salt-substitute seasoning mixture, for low-salt and low-fat—but succulent and savory—dishes. Don't feel you have to follow these recipes exactly. If you do change ingredients, adjust the seasonings, but don't add salt or any fats or oils.

Put your salt shaker back in the cabinet and take out your spice rack. Salt is often hidden in food products and not obvious, but your salt shaker is something that is easily seen and thus can be banished. On the next page is

Sparky Seasoning Mix

This recipe for a seasoning mix can be used instead of salt. It can be made in large quantities—just keep it in an airtight container in a cool dry place. Change the proportions to suit your taste.

White pepper	1½ teaspoons
Cayenne pepper	1 teaspoon
Black pepper	1 teaspoon
Onion powder	1 teaspoon
Garlic powder	1¼ teaspoons
Basil, dried	1 tablespoon
Thyme, dried	1½ tablespoons

Mix all ingredients together. Use this salt substitute in meat, poultry, fish, bean, or vegetable dishes. You can also use it to replace the salt in the salt shaker and use it at the table.

my favorite recipe for a salt substitute; you may want to change the spices or the proportions of each spice used.

The following recipes are grouped by type. Along with each group, you'll find general advice on buying and preparing the ingredients.

Grains

VEGGIE PASTA SAUCE

PER SERVING: CALORIES 100   TOTAL FAT 5 GRAMS   SATURATED FAT 1 GRAM
CHOLESTEROL 0 MILLIGRAMS   SODIUM 460 MILLIGRAMS

Olive oil	2 tablespoons
Onions, chopped	2 small
Zucchini, sliced	1¼ cups
Oregano, dried	1 tablespoon
Basil, dried	1 tablespoon
Tomato juice, low-salt	8 ounce can

> ## Tips About Breads, Cereals, Rice, and Pasta
>
> - Choose products made with whole grains as often as you can. Whole wheat, oatmeal, oat bran, rye, and pumpernickel breads are good choices, as are corn products, especially tortillas.
>
> - Cook pasta and rice without salt or fats, or with just a spray of vegetable oil on the pan. Try using unsalted broth or a low-salt vegetable juice to add flavor. Try flavored pastas found in many grocery stores, such as spinach, or herbed. Add nuts or beans for added texture and crunch, although since they add calories, use them in moderation. Brown rice has more flavor and fiber than ordinary polished white rice.
>
> - Make a pasta salad with last night's leftovers for lunch or dinner. If you need to, use a reduced-calorie mayonnaise salad dressing. Try making your own dressings with olive oil, vinegar, and seasonings.
>
> - When making pasta, rinse cooked pasta in hot water when it is removed from the stove. The hot water will wash away some of the starch in the pasta.

Tomato paste, low-salt	6 ounce can
Tomatoes, chopped	2 medium
Water	1 cup

In a medium skillet, heat oil. Sauté onions, garlic, zucchini for 5 minutes on medium heat.

Add remaining ingredients and simmer covered for 45 minutes. Serve over pasta.

MAKES 6 SERVINGS

Note: Omit the tomato juice and serve this recipe as a salsa dip with salt-free corn chips.

A dollop of this recipe can also be used to spice up a baked potato.

LASAGNA WITHOUT GUILT

PER SERVING: CALORIES 276 · TOTAL FAT 5 GRAMS   SATURATED FAT 2 GRAMS
CHOLESTEROL 11 MILLIGRAMS   SODIUM 380 MILLIGRAMS

Lasagna noodles, cooked in unsalted water	½ pound
Mozzarella cheese, skim milk, shredded	¾ cup
Cottage cheese, low-fat, low-salt	1½ cups
Parmesan cheese, low-fat, grated	¼ cup
Zucchini, raw, sliced	1½ cups
Tomato sauce, low-sodium	2½ cups
Basil, dried	2 teaspoons
Oregano, dried	2 teaspoons
Onion, chopped	¼ cup
Garlic, minced	1 clove
Black pepper	⅛ teaspoon

Preheat oven to 350°F. Lightly spray a 9 by 13 inch baking dish with vegetable oil. Set aside.

In a small bowl, combine ⅛ cup mozzarella cheese and 1 tablespoon Parmesan cheese with cottage cheese. Mix well and set aside.

In a medium bowl, combine remaining mozzarella and 1 tablespoon of Parmesan cheese. Mix well and set aside.

Combine tomato sauce with herbs, onion, garlic, and pepper. Spread a thin layer of tomato sauce on the bottom of the baking dish. Add about a third of the noodles in a single layer; spread half of the cottage cheese mixture on top. Add a layer of zucchini. Repeat layering. Add a thin coating of sauce. Top with the noodles, sauce, and reserved Mozzarella cheese mixture. Sprinkle on remaining 2 tablespoons Parmesan. Cover with aluminum foil.

Bake 30 to 40 minutes. Let stand 10 to 15 minutes. Cut into portions.

MAKES 6 SERVINGS

Spaghetti with a Gobble

PER SERVING: CALORIES 325 TOTAL FAT 9 GRAMS SATURATED FAT 6 GRAMS
CHOLESTEROL 15 MILLIGRAMS SODIUM 425 MILLIGRAMS

Olive oil	1 teaspoon
Turkey meat, ground	1 pound
Tomatoes, fresh or low-salt canned	1 can (28 ounces)
Green bell pepper, chopped	1 cup
Onion, chopped	1 cup
Garlic, minced	2 cloves
Oregano	1 teaspoon
Chili powder	1 teaspoon
Black pepper	1 teaspoon

Heat oil in a large skillet. Add turkey, cook for 5 minutes, stirring while cooking so meat does not stick to the bottom of the pan.

Drain fat.

Stir in tomatoes with their juice, green pepper, onion, garlic, oregano, and pepper.

Boil; turn down heat. Put lid on pan and cook on low heat for 15 minutes. Stir several times.

Take off cover; cook on low heat for 15 minutes.

In another pot, cook spaghetti in boiling water as directed.

Serve sauce over spaghetti.

MAKES 6 SERVINGS

Note: The meat can be made into small balls, and used in hero sandwiches.

Swimming with the Tuna

PER SERVING: CALORIES 195   TOTAL FAT 2 GRAMS   SATURATED FAT TRACE
CHOLESTEROL 13 MILLIGRAMS   SODIUM 170 MILLIGRAMS

Elbow macaroni, uncooked	¾ cup
Tuna, water-packed, drained	6½ ounce can
Celery, thinly sliced	½ cup
Seedless red grapes, halved	1 cup
Salad dressing, reduced-calorie mayonnaise-type	3 tablespoons

Cook macaroni, according to package directions, omitting salt. Drain completely.

Toss macaroni, tuna, celery, and grapes together.

Fold in salad dressing.

Serve warm or chilled.

MAKES 2 TO 3 SERVINGS

Note: This salad is a change from the typical tuna salad. It provides a serving of pasta and half a serving of fruit in addition to the tuna.

Vegetables

Hot Vegetable Bean Dip

PER TABLESPOON SERVING: CALORIES 15   TOTAL FAT TRACE   SATURATED FAT TRACE
CHOLESTEROL 0 MILLIGRAMS   SODIUM 55 MILLIGRAMS

Kidney beans, low-salt	15 ounce can
Drained bean liquid	3 tablespoons
Vinegar	1 tablespoon
Chili powder	1 teaspoon
Cumin, ground	⅛ teaspoon
Red pepper, ground	1 teaspoon
Onion, grated	2 teaspoons
Parsley, chopped	2 teaspoons

> ### Tips About Vegetables
>
> Raw and cooked vegetables provide needed dietary fiber. Raw vegetables have more vitamins than cooked. Try steaming; cook until they are still a bit crisp. Scrub your potatoes and eat them with their skins for more fiber. Beans and peas are inexpensive, and provide protein and fiber. They make a hearty soup or stew; or add them to rice dishes for a complete meal.
>
> Season vegetables with herbs, yogurt, and lemon juice. Limit butter, margarine, dressings, salt, and sauces. Canned vegetables are often high in sodium; try the no-salt-added products.

Drain kidney beans; set aside liquid.

Place drained beans, bean liquid, vinegar, cumin, and chili powder in blender. Blend until smooth.

Remove mixture from blender. Stir in hot pepper, onion, and parsley.

Chill thoroughly. Serve with sticks or wedges of crisp raw vegetables.

Makes about 1⅓ cups

Note: Substitute red, black, or white beans for kidney beans. My own favorite is navy beans; chickpeas are high in calories, but have a nice consistency for dips.

Herbal Zucchini Combo

PER SERVING: Calories 25   Total fat trace   Saturated fat trace
Cholesterol 0 milligrams   Sodium 10 milligrams

Water	2 tablespoons
Zucchini, thinly sliced	1 cup
Yellow squash, thinly sliced	1½ cups
Green pepper, cut into 2-inch strips	½ cup
Celery, cut into 2-inch strips	¼ cup
Onion, chopped	¼ cup
Caraway seed	½ teaspoon
Garlic powder	⅛ teaspoon
Tomato, cut into 8 wedges	1 medium

Heat water to a simmer in a large frying pan.

Add zucchini, squash, green pepper, celery, and onion. Cover and cook over moderate heat until vegetables are tender but still slightly crisp.

Sprinkle seasonings over vegetables. Add tomatoes; cook everything together about 2 minutes.

MAKES 4 SERVINGS

Note: This vegetable stew can be used as a sauce over rice, potatoes, or pasta.

BROCCOLI (OR OTHER VEGETABLE) SOUP

PER SERVING: CALORIES 110   TOTAL FAT 3 GRAMS   SATURATED FAT 2 GRAMS
CHOLESTEROL 9 MILLIGRAMS   SODIUM 250 MILLIGRAMS

Broccoli, chopped	1½ cups
Celery, diced	¼ cup
Onion, chopped	¼ cup
Chicken broth, unsalted	1 cup
Skim milk	2 cups
Cornstarch	2 tablespoons
Salt or substitute	dash
Black pepper	dash
Ground thyme	dash
Swiss or cheddar, low-fat cheese, shredded	¼ cup

Tips About Milk, Yogurt, and Cheese

Dairy foods are an important source of calcium, but they can add fat and sodium to your diet. Choose a lower fat and lower sodium version as often as you can. Consider skim milk, evaporated skim milk, low-fat or nonfat plain yogurt, whipped cottage cheese (high in sodium), part skim milk ricotta or other cheeses, low-fat processed cheese, and other low-fat cheeses. Generally, soft cheeses have fewer calories than hard cheeses.

Place vegetables and broth in saucepan. Bring to a boil, reduce heat, cover, and cook until vegetables are tender.

Mix milk, cornstarch, salt or substitute, pepper, and thyme; add to cooked vegetables. Cook, stirring, until soup is slightly thickened and mixture simmers.

Remove from heat. Add cheese and stir until melted.

MAKES 6 CUPS OR SMALL BOWLS

Note: Frozen broccoli, a 10 ounce package, may be used instead of fresh broccoli. Cauliflower or other vegetables can be used in place of broccoli. A cup can be partnered with a half sandwich for a hearty lunch or light supper.

ESCALLOPED CORN PUDDING

PER SERVING: CALORIES 230   TOTAL FAT 6 GRAMS   SATURATED FAT 40 GRAMS
CHOLESTEROL 70 MILLIGRAMS   SODIUM 250 MILLIGRAMS

Creamed corn, low-salt	*1 can*
Egg white	*1*
Milk, low-fat	*⅔ cup*
Cracker crumbs	*½ cup*
Cheese, low-fat white, shredded	*¼ cup*
Whipped butter	*2 teaspoons*
Black pepper	*dash*
Nutmeg	*dash*

Preheat oven to 325°F.

Mix all ingredients in a large baking dish. Bake for 30 minutes, or until crisp and brown.

MAKES 6 SERVINGS

Terrific Taco Salad

PER SERVING: CALORIES 220   TOTAL FAT 12 GRAMS   SATURATED FAT 8 GRAMS
CHOLESTEROL 45 MILLIGRAMS   SODIUM 320 MILLIGRAMS

Lettuce, shredded	1½ cups
Tomatoes, chopped	¾ cup
Kidney beans, canned, drained	1 cup
Green bell pepper, chopped	½ cup
Cooked chicken, chopped	1 cup
Salsa, low-sodium	½ cup
Taco cups, commercial or homemade	4 small taco cups or shells
Cheddar cheese, low-fat, shredded	½ cup
Sour cream, low-fat	½ cup

Toss the lettuce, tomatoes, beans, pepper, and chicken together in large bowl. Add salsa.

Spoon the mixture into the taco shells; top with sprinkled cheddar cheese and a dollop of sour cream.

MAKES 4 LARGE TACOS

Tips About Beef, Pork, Chicken, and Fish

Always select lean cuts of meat. Round steak instead of sirloin in beef. For any kind of meat, choose a steak rather than a chop, because a loin cut is usually lower in fat. White breast meat, which is low in fat, in place of dark thigh meat in poultry. Remember to remove as much fat as possible before cooking, and skin chicken or other poultry before cooking. Avoid rich sauces when serving fish; broiled or steamed fish is low in fat. Use nonstick pans or spray pan with a light oil when cooking meat. Tip: Bake any meat loaf in an extra large pan or use a rack so the fat drains to the sides of the pan.

Meat, Poultry, and Fish

SWEET AND SOUR ROAST PORK

PER SERVING: CALORIES 450   TOTAL FAT 10 GRAMS   SATURATED FAT 8 GRAMS
CHOLESTEROL 180 MILLIGRAMS   SODIUM 610 MILLIGRAMS

Salt	dash
Black pepper	½ teaspoon
Pork fillet, uncut	2 pounds
Onion, small, minced	½ cup
Green bell pepper, minced	½ cup
Tomato, chopped	½ cup
Olive oil	1 tablespoon
Vinegar, white	2 tablespoons
Honey	2 tablespoons
Mustard, ground	1 tablespoon
Potatoes, round white	4 small
Parsley, minced	1 teaspoon

Preheat oven to 375°F.

Sprinkle salt and pepper on the pork; coat the surface with a mixture of vegetables, oil, vinegar, honey, and mustard.

Place the pork in a roasting pan, uncovered. Place potatoes around the pork.

Place in oven and roast for two hours. (Cook until there is no pink, or use a meat thermometer.)

Thinly slice the pork, serve without the gravy. Add roasted potatoes. Garnish with parsley.

MAKE 6 SERVINGS

Note: Refrigerate the leftovers. When the fat hardens, chip it off with a spoon. Use the pork in sandwiches for lunch or supper.

"Lite" Beef Stroganoff

PER SERVING: CALORIES 275   TOTAL FAT 6 GRAMS   SATURATED FAT 2 GRAMS
CHOLESTEROL 71 MILLIGRAMS   SODIUM 325 MILLIGRAMS

Beef, boneless round steak, trimmed	¾ pound
Mushrooms, fresh	¼ pound
Onion, sliced	½ cup
Beef broth, low-salt	½ cup
Water	½ cup
Catsup, low-salt	1 tablespoon
Black pepper	⅛ teaspoon
Flour	2 tablespoons
Buttermilk	1 cup
Noodles, cooked, unsalted	2 cups

MAKES 4 SERVINGS

Slice steak across the grain into thin strips, about ⅛ inch wide and 3 inches long. (It is easier to cut thin slices of meat if it is partially frozen.) Wash and slice mushrooms.

Cook beef strips, mushrooms, and onion in nonstick skillet until beef is lightly browned.

Add broth, water, catsup, and pepper. Cover and simmer until beef is tender, about 45 minutes.

Mix flour with about ¼ cup of the buttermilk until smooth; add remaining buttermilk. Stir into beef mixture. Cook, stirring constantly, until thickened.

Serve over noodles.

MAKES 4 SERVINGS

Note: The modifications in a traditional Stroganoff recipe have saved about 240 calories. The same recipe can be served over cooked rice.

Oriental Beef and Vegetable Stir-fry

PER SERVING: CALORIES 145   TOTAL FAT 4 GRAMS   SATURATED FAT 1 GRAM
CHOLESTEROL 44 MILLIGRAMS   SODIUM 300 MILLIGRAMS

Beef, round steak, boneless	*¾ pound*
Vegetable oil	*1 teaspoon*
Carrots, sliced	*½ cup*
Celery, chopped	*½ cup*
Onion, sliced	*½ cup*
Soy sauce	*dash*
Garlic powder	*⅛ teaspoon*
Black pepper	*dash*
Zucchini, cut into strips	*2 cups*
Cornstarch	*1 tablespoon*
Water	*¼ cup*

Trim all the visible fat from steak. Slice steak across the grain into thin strips about ⅛ inch wide and 3 inches long. (Note: Partially frozen meat is easier to slice.)

Heat oil in skillet. Add carrots, celery, onion, and seasonings. Cover and cook until carrots are slightly tender.

Add squash; cook until vegetables are tender-crisp.

Add beef strips and stir-fry over high heat, turning pieces constantly until beef is no longer red or even pink—about 3 to 5 minutes. Reduce heat.

Mix cornstarch and water until smooth; add slowly to beef mixture. Cook until thickened and vegetables are coated with a thin glaze.

MAKES 4 SERVINGS, ABOUT ¾ CUP EACH

Note: Shrimp or small bits of crab meat can be used instead of beef. Beware of using too much soy sauce, as it is very high in sodium.

Oriental Chicken and Vegetable Stir-fry

PER SERVING: CALORIES 140   TOTAL FAT 2 GRAMS   SATURATED FAT TRACE
CHOLESTEROL 51 MILLIGRAMS   SODIUM 320 MILLIGRAMS

Use 3 boneless, skinless chicken breast halves (about 12 ounces of raw chicken) in place of beef in previous recipe. Slice chicken into thin strips. Chicken should be cooked until thoroughly done or no longer pink.

MAKES 4 SERVINGS, ABOUT ¾ CUP EACH

Note: The trick in Oriental cooking is to make it fast. Keep the food moving in the pan. This recipe can also be steamed, for a really healthy (low-fat) version.

Chicken and Spanish Rice

PER SERVING: CALORIES 406   TOTAL FAT 6 GRAMS   SATURATED FAT 2 GRAMS
CHOLESTEROL 75 MILLIGRAMS   SODIUM 367 MILLIGRAMS

Onion, chopped	*1 cup*
Green bell pepper, chopped	*¾ cup*
Olive oil	*2 teaspoons*
Tomato sauce, low-sodium	*1 cup*
Parsley, chopped	*1 teaspoon*
Black pepper	*¼ teaspoon*
Garlic, minced	*1½ teaspoons*
White rice, cooked in unsalted water	*5 cups*
Chicken breast, skinless, cooked, chopped	*3¼ cups*

In a large skillet sauté onion and green pepper in oil for 5 minutes on medium heat.

Add tomato sauce and spices. Heat through. Add cooked rice and chicken and heat through.

MAKES 5 SERVINGS, ABOUT 1½ CUPS EACH

CHICKEN SALAD

PER SERVING: CALORIES 183 TOTAL FAT 7 GRAMS SATURATED FAT 2 GRAMS
CHOLESTEROL 78 MILLIGRAMS SODIUM 200 MILLIGRAMS

Chicken breast, skinless, cooked, cubed	3½ cups
Celery, chopped	¼ cup
Lemon juice	1 tablespoon
Onion powder	½ teaspoon
Soy sauce	dash

Combine all ingredients in a large mixing bowl. Gently toss and fold. Serve the salad on lettuce leaves and garnish with orange wedges.

MAKES 5 SERVINGS

TUSCANY CHICKEN

PER SERVING: CALORIES 280 TOTAL FAT 3 GRAMS SATURATED FAT 1 GRAM
CHOLESTEROL 68 MILLIGRAMS SODIUM 320 MILLIGRAMS

Chicken breasts, skinned	4
Olive oil	1 teaspoon
Spaghetti, thin, broken in pieces	4 ounces
Onion, cut in wedges	1 small
Green bell pepper, cut in strips	1 small
Garlic, instant minced	⅛ teaspoon
Oregano leaves	1 teaspoon
Salt	dash
Black pepper	⅛ teaspoon
Bay leaf	1
Tomatoes	3 small
Water	¼ cup
Parsley, chopped	1 tablespoon

Place chicken breasts between sheets of plastic wrap. Pound with a heavy weight until about ½ inch thick.

Heat oil in skillet. Brown chicken breasts on each side.

Add spaghetti, onion, and pepper strips around chicken. Sprinkle garlic and seasoning over the dish.

Cut tomatoes into large pieces and pour tomatoes and water over top of chicken.

Bring to a boil; reduce heat, cover, and cook until chicken and spaghetti are done, about 15 minutes.

Remove bay leaf. Garnish with parsley.

MAKES 4 SERVINGS

Note: Serve with a spinach salad and a small amount of reduced-calorie dressing and garlic bread. (Garlic bread: a small amount of olive oil and dash of garlic powder on a crusty bread.)

TUSCANY TURKEY

PER SERVING: CALORIES 275   TOTAL FAT 8 GRAMS   SATURATED FAT TRACE
CHOLESTEROL 70 MILLIGRAMS   SODIUM 305 MILLIGRAMS

Use 1 pound raw turkey breast fillets or tenderloins in place of chicken in previous recipe.

BROILED SESAME FISH

PER SERVING: CALORIES 110   TOTAL FAT 3 GRAMS   SATURATED FAT TRACE
CHOLESTEROL 46 MILLIGRAMS   SODIUM 155 MILLIGRAMS

Cod fillets, fresh or frozen	*1 pound*
Olive oil	*1 teaspoon*
Lemon juice	*1 tablespoon*
Dried tarragon leaves	*1 teaspoon*
Salt	*dash*
Black pepper	*dash*
Sesame seeds	*1 tablespoon*
Parsley, chopped	*1 tablespoon*

Cut fish into four portions. (Fresh fish is always best; thaw frozen fish in refrigerator overnight or defrost in microwave.)

Place fish on a broiler pan lined with foil; brush with oil. Mix lemon juice, tarragon leaves, salt, and pepper. Pour over fish.

Sprinkle sesame seeds evenly over fish.

Broil until fish flakes easily when tested with a fork. Garnish with parsley.

MAKES 4 PORTIONS

Note: This fish recipe is quick, easy, and low-fat. Almost any flat fish will be delicious with this recipe. Trout is wonderful.

DIZZY DILL FISH

PER SERVING: CALORIES 90   TOTAL FAT 2 GRAMS   SATURATED FAT TRACE
CHOLESTEROL 45 MILLIGRAMS   SODIUM 130 MILLIGRAMS

Fish fillets	1 pound (4 pieces)
Lemon juice	1 tablespoon
Dried dill weed	¼ teaspoon
Salt	dash
Black pepper	dash

Separate fish into fillets or pieces.

Place fish in heated nonstick skillet, and spray with oil. Sprinkle with lemon juice and seasonings.

Cover and cook over moderate heat until fish flakes when tested with a fork.

MAKES 4 SERVINGS

Note: Try this recipe with catfish fillets; they have fewer calories. The dill and lemon juice provide moist flavor, without butter. Serve with carrots, celery, rice, potatoes. This dinner is so low in calories, you can splurge on dessert. Fish fillets can be cooked in a microwave oven; cook at medium power.

Spicy Baked Salmon

PER SERVING: CALORIES 135–160   TOTAL FAT 7 GRAMS   SATURATED FAT 4 GRAMS
CHOLESTEROL 75 MILLIGRAMS   SODIUM 100 MILLIGRAMS

Salmon fillets	1 pound (4 pieces)
Olive oil	1 tablespoon
Sparky Seasoning Mix (p. 284)	1 teaspoon

Follow the directions for Dizzy Dill Fish.

MAKES 4 SERVINGS

Fruits and Desserts

Apple Crisp

PER SERVING: CALORIES 235   TOTAL FAT 9 GRAMS   SATURATED FAT 2 GRAMS
CHOLESTEROL 0 MILLIGRAMS   SODIUM 105 MILLIGRAMS

Tart apples, pared, sliced	4 cups
Water	¼ cup
Lemon juice	1 tablespoon
Brown sugar, packed	¼ cup
Whole wheat flour	¼ cup
Old-fashioned rolled oats	¼ cup
Ground cinnamon	¼ teaspoon
Ground nutmeg	¼ teaspoon
Low-calorie butter substitute	2 tablespoons

Preheat oven to 350°F.

Place apples in 8 by 2 inch baking pan. (A glass baking pan is easier to clean.)

Mix water and lemon juice, pour over apples. Mix sugar, flour, oats, and spices.

Add butter to dry mixture; mix until crumbly. Sprinkle crumbly mixture evenly over apples.

Bake until apples are tender to a fork probe and the topping is lightly browned.

MAKES 4 SERVINGS

JIGGLING MOLD

PER SERVING: CALORIES 320   TOTAL FAT TRACE   SATURATED FAT TRACE
     CHOLESTEROL TRACE   SODIUM 230 MILLIGRAMS

Strawberry gelatin, low-fat	2 3-ounce packages
Boiling water	2 cups
Strawberries, frozen sliced	2 10-ounce packages
Pineapple, crushed, unsweetened, well drained	3½ cups
Bananas, sliced	2
Cottage cheese, low-calorie, low-salt	1 small container, 8 ounces

Dissolve the strawberry gelatin in the hot water.

Add the strawberries, stir until thawed. Add the crushed pineapple and the bananas.

Pour half of the mixture into a mold, and chill until firm. Remove from

---

Tips About Fruits and Desserts

Desserts are not forbidden. Finish your meals with fruit. The natural sweetness will leave you with a satisfied feeling. Serve fruit at room temperature for a sweeter flavor. All fruits have some fiber, vitamins, and minerals. Fresh or frozen fruits are best. Blend fresh, frozen, or canned fruit with low-calorie milk, and freeze to a slush for a smoothie treat.

Bake or broil apples, pears, or peaches. Bananas, rich in potassium, can be sprinkled with cinnamon or nutmeg.

Rice cakes are the best treat you can have. They can be made into cookies by placing a small piece of chocolate (the size of half a chocolate kiss) on top of each cake and melting in a microwave.

the refrigerator and spread with the cottage cheese. Pour the remaining gelatin and fruit mixture on top.

Chill until firm. Remove mold by turning out on chilled plate. Garnish with fresh fruit.

MAKES 6–8 SERVINGS

BRAN APPLE BARS

PER BAR: CALORIES 110   TOTAL FAT 4 GRAMS   SATURATED FAT 1 GRAM
CHOLESTEROL TRACE   SODIUM 120 MILLIGRAMS

Whole bran cereal, unsweetened	1 cup
Skim milk	½ cup
Flour	1 cup
Baking powder	1 teaspoon
Cinnamon, ground	½ teaspoon
Nutmeg	¼ teaspoon
Margarine	⅓ cup
Brown sugar, packed	½ cup
Egg whites	2
Apples, cored, pared, and chopped	1 cup

Preheat oven to 350°F. Grease a 9 inch square pan.

Soak bran in milk until all milk is absorbed.

Mix dry ingredients, and set aside.

Beat margarine and sugar together until creamy. Add egg whites and beat well. Stir in apples and bran mixture. Add dry ingredients; mix well.

Pour into greased pan, bake until a toothpick inserted in the center comes out clean.

Cool slightly. Cut into bars while still warm.

MAKES 16 BARS

Note: Look for low-sodium baking powder. You can adapt this recipe to work with pears; use dried fruits in place of the brown sugar for flavor and additional fiber.

Zucchini Bread

PER SLICE: CALORIES 110   TOTAL FAT 4 GRAMS   SATURATED FAT 1 GRAM
CHOLESTEROL TRACE   SODIUM 290 MILLIGRAMS

Whole wheat flour	1 cup
All-purpose flour	1 cup
Baking powder	1½ teaspoons
Cinnamon, ground	1 teaspoon
Baking soda	¼ teaspoon
Salt	dash
Egg whites	3
Sugar	½ cup
Oil, corn or vegetable	⅓ cup
Vanilla	1½ teaspoons
Zucchini, coarsely shredded, lightly packed	2 cups

Preheat oven to 350°F. Spray or grease loaf pan with vegetable oil.

Mix dry ingredients, except sugar.

Beat egg whites until frothy, Add sugar, oil, and vanilla. Continue beating for several minutes.

Add dry ingredients and zucchini; mix until moistened.

Pour into loaf pan.

Bake 40 minutes or until toothpick inserted in center comes out clean.

Turn out, and cool on rack.

MAKES 18 SMALL SLICES

Note: Bananas or yams can be used instead of zucchini; adjust the cinnamon or add some nutmeg or other flavorings.

OATMEAL-RAISIN COOKIES

PER COOKIE: CALORIES 55   TOTAL FAT 2 GRAMS   SATURATED FAT 2 GRAMS
CHOLESTEROL TRACE   SODIUM 60 MILLIGRAMS

All-purpose flour	1 cup
Baking powder	1 teaspoon
Ground allspice	1 teaspoon
Salt	dash
Margarine	½ cup
Sugar	½ cup
Egg whites	2
Old-fashioned rolled oats	1 cup
Applesauce, unsweetened	1 cup
Raisins	½ cup

Preheat oven to 375°F. Lightly spray or grease baking sheets.

Mix dry ingredients together, except oats. Set aside.

Beat margarine and sugar until creamy. Add egg whites; beat well.

Add dry ingredients.

Stir in oats, applesauce, and raisins. Mix well.

Drop by level tablespoonsful onto greased baking sheet.

Bake until lightly browned and edges are crisp. Cool on a rack.

MAKES 5 DOZEN SMALL COOKIES

Low-Pressure Shopping

You can food-shop and buy most of your favorite foods yet still stay within your DASH or antihypertensive diet. Just choose the products that are right for you. It would be foolish and a waste of money, besides being painful, to buy shoes that aren't the right size or don't fit the contours of your foot. The same care should be extended to food shopping. Choose food items that are right for your body.

Use the handy guide below to shop for a variety of blood-pressure-pleasing foods. By eating a variety of foods each day you will get the nutrients you need. Remember to read the food labels, which will give you the nutritional information of each food product you buy. Look for products that say low-fat, lean, or light. Also, look for low-salt, salt-free products. But don't take those words at face value—you still must read the labels. The U.S. government has defined these words to help consumers find hypertension-happy foods that contain less saturated fat, cholesterol, and sodium.

Buy Right

Here is a guide to the types of foods to look for and to buy. Don't go shopping when you are hungry; it will make foods that aren't right for you seem especially tempting.

MEAT, POULTRY, FISH, SHELLFISH

Choose lean cuts of meat with fat; trim meat before cooking.

Beef—round, top loin, sirloin, chuck arm, pot roast; all well trimmed

Lamb—leg shank, fore shank, leg, loin; well trimmed with the fat drained

Pork—tenderloin, sirloin, top loin; canned ham is often heavily salted

Veal—cutlets, ground, shoulder, sirloin, rib roast

Chicken and turkey—skinless, broiled or baked; fried chicken and duck or goose are high in fat

Seafood—flat freshwater fish and fresh or frozen ocean fish

- If you want a hamburger, before eating it, press it between the top and bottom of the hamburger roll to remove excess fat; discard the roll.

- Many deli meats have been created from seasoned turkey. Some of these imitations mimic the real thing, and they are usually low-fat, but many are high in sodium. Make your choice after reading the labels. Most fresh meat, poultry, and fish is low in sodium. Most cured and processed meats, such as hot dogs, sausage, and luncheon meats, are high in sodium, which is used as a preservative.

DAIRY PRODUCTS

Skim or 1 percent fat milk

Nonfat or low-fat yogurt

Cheese with 3 grams of fat or less per ounce

Low-fat or nonfat sour cream

• Look for low-sodium as well as low-fat cheese; generally the softer the cheese, the lower the fat content. However, cottage cheese is very high in sodium. The sodium content of milk and milk products varies. Lowest are milk and yogurt. In terms of sodium, natural cheese contains some, then comes processed cheeses, cheese foods, and cheese spreads.

EGGS

Egg whites only

Cholesterol-free or cholesterol-reduced egg substitutes

• You can eat eggs in moderation.

FATS AND OILS

Unsaturated vegetable oils: corn, olive, canola, sesame, soybean, sunflower, safflower

Soft margarine made with unsaturated fats listed above

Reduced or nonfat mayonnaise

• Salad bars are not as low-fat or good for you as you may think; just a tablespoon of dressing with a creamy or mayonnaise base makes a salad higher in calories.

FRUITS

Fresh or frozen fruits

Canned (low-sugar, or no sugar added) and fruit preserved in its own juice, with no sugar added

VEGETABLES

Fresh or frozen vegetables; canned vegetables have sodium added.

Tofu (comes in small cakes), low-salt—use as a meat substitute or extender

• Most canned vegetables, vegetable juices, and frozen vegetables with sauce are higher in sodium than fresh. Avoid any cheese sauce on your vegetables. Cook vegetables without adding salt, it will make a big difference in your sodium consumption.

BEVERAGES

Caffeine-free drinks

Fruit drinks or punches with no sugar added, or concentrated fruit juice, which can be thinned to suit your taste by adding water

- Many sodas have salt added, including those that are low-calorie or caffeine-free.

BREADS, CEREALS, PASTA, RICE AND GRAINS, DRY PEAS AND BEANS

Breads, white or whole grain (whole grain is best; it has more fiber), pitas, bagels, English muffins, sandwich buns, dinner rolls

Rice cakes

Corn tortillas (avoid wheat, which has shortening)

Pretzels, crackers like matzo, bread sticks, rye crackers, low-salt, low-fat

Pancakes, waffles, low-fat

Muffins, low-fat

Hot cereals, most cold cereals, low-fat

Rice, barley, bulgur

Dry peas and beans

Pasta

- Avoid biscuits or croissants, which are high in sodium and fat.

SWEETS AND SNACKS

Nonfat and low-fat frozen desserts like sherbet, sorbet, Italian ice, frozen yogurt, frozen fruit juice bars

Freeze grapes or melon balls

Top low-calorie angel food cake with fresh or slushy frozen fruit

Low-fat or nonfat baked goods like brownies, cakes, cupcakes, pastries, fig or other fruit bars, vanilla or lemon wafers, graham crackers, ginger snaps

Jelly beans, hard candy, fruit leather

Plain popcorn, pretzels, baked salt-free chips

A Healthy Way to Adapt Convenience Staples

You can reduce fat and sodium in the boxed products you use, such as macaroni and cheese. Just follow the chart below:

Mix	Changes	Serving size	Fat saved per serving	Sodium saved per serving
Macaroni and cheese	Omit salt Use low-fat milk Reduce margarine	¾ cup	6 g	265 mg
Seasoned rice	Reduce margarine by half	½ cup	2 g	20 mg
Bread stuffing	Reduce margarine by half	½ cup	4 g	45 mg
Scalloped or gratin potatoes	Use low-fat milk Reduce margarine	½ cup	2 g	20 mg

Cook It Right

Buying the freshest, lowest calorie, and lowest sodium foods is a good start on your HBP diet, but food is often no better than the way you cook it. Here are some easy cooking tips to reduce saturated fat, cholesterol, and sodium as much as possible:

Before cooking meat, poultry, and fish trim fat from meat; remove the skin and fat from poultry. If you buy tuna or other canned fish, look for the variety that's packed in water. If you are not sure how salty the fish is, you can put the fish in a sieve and rinse it in cold water.

Changes in your cooking style can also lower fat and sodium intake. Bake, broil, microwave, poach, or roast instead of frying. When you do fry, use a nonstick pan and only a light coating of nonstick cooking spray. You can make your own oil sprayer by cleaning a small spray bottle and filling it with olive oil; then spray just a little on the bottom and sides of the pan before cooking.

When you roast meat or make meat loaf, place the meat on a rack or a larger than usual pan so the fat can drip away. When a recipe calls for ground meat, brown the meat and drain the liquid fat well before adding the other ingredients. When you baste meats and poultry, use fruit juice, lemon juice, or broth instead of the fatty drippings.

Sauces, soups, and casseroles can either be a fat trap or a nutritious focus for your meal. After making sauces or soups, cool them in the refrigerator and skim the hardened fat from the top. When making casseroles with cheese, try lower fat cheese. Or use less of the cheese than the recipe calls for. If you use a sharp-flavored cheese you won't taste the difference.

When you make creamed soups or white sauces, use skim, 1 percent, or evaporated skim milk instead of 2 percent milk, whole milk, or cream. To make a low-fat sauce, thicken it with cornstarch or flour.

Make main dishes with pasta, rice, or dry peas and beans. If you add meat, use small pieces just for flavoring instead of as the main ingredient.

Seasoning and condiments can make a meal delightful. Use small amounts of lean meat instead of salt pork or fatback, to flavor vegetables while cooking. Flavor-cook vegetables with herbs or butter-flavored seasoning instead of butter or margarine.

Use herbs, spices, and no-salt seasoning to bring out the flavor of dishes. Garlic and garlic powder, onion or onion powder are a cook's best friend. Use salt sparingly in cooking and use less salt at the table. Reduce the amount a little each day until no salt is used. Limit or delete entirely salty condiments like olives and pickles.

Convenience foods are attractive, and make sense when you have a hurried day, and for those times when you don't feel like cooking. Check the Nutrition Facts to choose frozen dinners and pizzas that are lower in saturated fat, cholesterol, and sodium. Make sure the dinners have vegetables, fruits, and grains—or add them on the side. Better yet: Use your own convenience foods—low-fat casseroles and soups that you have cooked ahead of time and have ready frozen in small batches.

Use fewer sauces, mixes, and instant products, including flavored rices, pastas, and cereal, which usually have added salt. Use vegetables that are fresh, frozen without sauce, or canned with no salt added.

Serving sizes should be small because, obviously, the larger the serving, the more salt and fat you will consume. Recognizing portion size is an important part of being in control of what you eat. Here are some tips to help you recognize a portion size: Look at your hand; a piece of meat the size of the palm of a small hand is about 3 ounces. To find out how much food you are serving yourself and your family at meals, try dishing it up with a measuring cup; after a few times, it will be easy to judge the size of the portions. Every time you see a small cookie, about the size of the president's picture on a paper bill, you should realize that it is at least 50 calories, probably more. In general, a small slice of cake, without the icing, is lower in calories than pies or pastry.

To get your daily dose of fiber eat at least six servings of whole grains (bread, cereals, pasta, rice) daily. Check food labels for how much fiber is in each. One serving of fiber is:

½ cup fruit

¾ cup juice (fruit juice is high in calories)

½ cup cooked vegetables

1 cup leafy salad vegetables

1 medium apple

1 slice of bread

1 ounce of dry cereal

½ cup cooked cereal, rice, or pasta

How to Modify Your Favorite Recipes

Lots of special cookbooks and recipe booklets can help you prepare foods that will lower the fat, saturated fat, cholesterol, and sodium when you cook. You can also send a postcard to: The National Heart, Lung, and Blood Institute Information Center, P.O. Box 30105, Bethesda, MD 20824-0105. They have booklets and other materials that will help you maintain a low-sodium, low-fat diet.

However, suppose you have favorite family recipes you have used for years. Or suppose you would like to enjoy special holiday foods. Just cut down as much as possible on the high-fat, high-sodium ingredients and substitute ingredients lower in saturated fat, cholesterol, and sodium. Here are some recipe substitutions that will minimize any changes in texture, consistency, and flavor:

Healthy Ingredient Substitutions

Instead of	Use
Whole milk	Skim or 1 percent milk
Evaporated milk	Evaporated skim milk
Light cream	Equal amounts of 1 percent milk and evaporated skim milk
Heavy cream	Evaporated skim milk
1 cup butter	1 cup soft margarine or ⅔ cup vegetable oil
Shortening or lard	Soft margarine
Mayonnaise or salad dressing	Nonfat or light mayonnaise or salad dressing; mustard in sandwiches
1 whole egg	¼ cup egg substitute or 2 egg whites
Cheese	Lower fat, lower sodium cheese
Cream cheese	Nonfat or reduced-calorie cream cheese
Sour cream	Nonfat or low-fat sour cream or yogurt
Fat for greasing pan	Nonstick cooking spray
1 ounce baking chocolate	3 tablespoons cocoa powder plus 1 tablespoon vegetable oil
Regular bouillon or broth	Low-sodium bouillon or broth
Fatback, neck bone, or ham	Skinless chicken or turkey bones
Pork bacon	Turkey bacon, lean ham, or Canadian bacon—only if low in sodium
Pork sausage	Ground skinless turkey breast with added herbs to taste
Ground beef and pork	Ground skinless turkey breast with added egg white for texture and herbs for seasonings

Now you are ready to put all of these do's and don'ts to work. Using the recipe substitutions here, or others that you develop, you'll soon be modifying your own favorite recipes, and you'll be able to eat your favorite dishes and share them with your friends and family.

Best Wishes for a Long and Happy Life

Living with hypertension requires that you become aware of yourself—your body, your diet, and your emotions and how they affect your blood pressure. Some of my patients have found that they feel better and are more able to enjoy life after they learned they have high blood pressure. This is because they have taken control of their habits, and feel excited and interested in life. I hope that is also your discovery.

Sodium in Foods

SODIUM IN FOODS (in Milligrams)

MEAT, POULTRY, FISH, AND SHELLFISH

Fresh meat (including lean cuts of beef, pork, lamb and veal), poultry, fin fish, cooked, 3 oz . . . . less than 90
Shellfish, 3 oz 100–325
Tuna, canned, 3 oz 300
*Sausage, 2 oz 515
*Bologna, 2 oz 535
*Frankfurter, 1½ oz 560
Boiled ham, 2 oz 750
Lean ham, 3 oz 1,025

EGGS

Egg white, 1 55
*Whole egg, 1 65
Egg substitute, ¼ cup = 1 egg 80–120

DAIRY PRODUCTS

MILK

*Whole milk, 1 cup 120
Skim or 1% milk, 1 cup 125
Buttermilk (salt added), 1 cup 260

CHEESE

*NATURAL CHEESE:

   *Swiss cheese, 1 oz 75
   *Cheddar cheese, 1 oz 175
   *Blue cheese, 1 oz 395
Low-fat cheese, 1 oz 150
*Process cheese and cheese spreads, 1 oz 340–450
Lower sodium and fat versions . . . . read the label
*Cottage cheese (regular), ½ cup 455
*Cottage cheese (low-fat), ½ cup 460

YOGURT

*Yogurt, whole milk, plain, 8 oz 105
Yogurt, fruited or flavored, low-fat or nonfat, 8 oz 120–150
Yogurt, nonfat or low-fat, plain, 8 oz 160–175

VEGETABLES

Fresh or frozen vegetables, or no-salt-added canned (cooked without salt), ½ cup . . . . Less than 70
Vegetables, canned, no sauce, ½ cup 55–470
*Vegetables, canned or frozen with sauce, ½ cup . . . . Read the label
Tomato juice, canned, ¾ cup 660

BREADS, CEREALS, RICE, PASTA, DRY PEAS AND BEANS

BREADS AND CRACKERS

Bread, 1 slice 110–175
English muffin, ½ 130
Bagel, ½ 190
Cracker, saltine type, 5 squares 195
*Baking powder biscuit, 1 305

CEREALS

READY-TO-EAT:

Shredded wheat, ¾ cup . . . . less than 5
Puffed wheat and rice cereals, 1½ to 1¾ cups . . . . less than 5
Granola-type cereals, ½ cup 5–25
Ring and nugget cereals, 1 cup 170–330
Flaked cereals, ⅔ to 1 cup 170–360

COOKED:

Cooked cereal (unsalted), ½ cup . . . . less than 5
Instant cooked cereal, 1 packet = ¾ cup 180

PASTA AND RICE

Cooked rice and pasta (unsalted), ½ cup . . . . less than 10
*Flavored rice mix, cooked, ½ cup 250–390

PEAS AND BEANS

Peanut butter, unsalted, 2 tbsp . . . . less than 5
Peanut butter, 2 tbsp 150

Dry beans, home-cooked
(unsalted), or no-salt-added, canned,
½ cup . . . . less than 5
Dry beans, plain, canned, ½ cup 350–590
*Dry beans, canned with
added fat or meat, ½ cup 425–630

FRUITS

Fruits (fresh, frozen,
canned), ½ cup . . . . less than 10

FATS AND OILS

Oil, 1 tbsp. 0
Butter, unsalted, 1 tsp. 1
Butter, salted, 1 tsp. 25
Margarine, unsalted, 1 tsp . . . . less than 5
Margarine, salted, 1 tsp 50
Imitation mayonnaise, 1 tbsp 75
*Mayonnaise, 1 tbsp. 80
Prepared salad dressings, low-calorie,
2 tbsp 50–310
*Prepared salad dressings,
2 tbsp 210–440

SNACKS

POPCORN, CHIPS, AND NUTS
Unsalted nuts, ¼ cup. . . . . less than 5
Salted nuts, ¼ cup. 185
*Unsalted potato chips and corn chips,
1 cup . . . . less than 5

*Salted potato chips and corn chips,
1 cup 170–285
Unsalted popcorn, 2½ cups. . . . . less than 10
Salted popcorn, 2½ cups. 330

CANDY
Jelly beans, 10 large 5
*Milk chocolate bar, 1 oz. 25

FROZEN DESSERTS
*Ice cream, ½ cup. 35–50
Frozen yogurt, low-fat or nonfat,
½ cup 40–55
Ice milk, ½ cup 55–60

CONDIMENTS

Mustard, chili sauce, hot sauce,
1 tsp 35-65
Catsup, steak sauce, 1 tbsp 100–230
Salsa, tartar sauce, 2 tbsp 200–315
Salt, ⅛ tsp. 390
Pickles, 5 slices . . . . 280—460
Soy sauce, lower sodium, 1 tbsp 600
Soy sauce, 1 tbsp 1,030

CONVENIENCE FOODS

**Canned and dehydrated
soups, 1 cup 600–1,300
**Lower sodium versions . . . . Read label
***Canned and frozen main dishes,
8 oz. 500–1,570
***Lower sodium versions . . . . Read label

Choices are higher in saturated fat, cholesterol, or both.

**Creamy soups are higher in saturated fat and cholesterol.*

***Limit main dishes that have ingredients higher in saturated fat, cholesterol, or both.*

Source: Adapted from Home and Garden Bulletin 253-7, United States Department of Agriculture, July 1993.

A Week with the DASH Diet

Here is a week of menus from the DASH eating plan. The menus are based on 2,000 calories a day—serving sizes should be increased or decreased for other caloric levels. Also, to ease the calculations, some of the serving sizes have been rounded off.

DAY 1		SERVINGS PROVIDED							
Food	Amount	Grains	Vegetables	Fruits	Dairy foods	Meat, poultry, & fish	Nuts, seeds, & dry beans	Fats & oils	Sweets
BREAKFAST									
apple juice	1 cup			1½					
bran cereal, ready-to-eat	⅔ cup	1							
raisins	2 tbsp			½					
fat-free milk	1 cup				1				
whole wheat bread	1 slice	1							
soft margarine	1½ tsp							1½	
LUNCH									
chicken sandwich:									
chicken breast, no skin	3 oz					1			
American cheese, reduced-fat	2 slices (1½ oz)				1				
leaf lettuce	2 large leaves		½						
tomato	2 slices (¼" thick)		½						
light mayonnaise	1 tbsp							1	
whole wheat bread	2 slices	2							
apple	1 medium			1					
DINNER									
veggie pasta sauce*	¾ cup		1½						
spaghetti, cooked	1 cup	2							
Parmesan cheese	4 tbsp				1				
green beans, cooked	½ cup		1						
spinach salad:									
spinach, raw	1 cup		1						
mushrooms, raw	¼ cup		¼						
croutons	2 tbsp	¼							
Italian dressing, low-fat	2 tbsp							1	
dinner roll	1 medium	1							
frozen yogurt, low-fat	½ cup				½				
SNACKS									
orange juice	1 cup			1½					
banana	1 large			1½					
TOTALS		7¼	4¾	6	3½	1	0	3½	0

PER DAY: 1,995 calories, 50 g total fat, 15 g saturated fat, 124 mg cholesterol, 458 mg magnesium, 4,254 mg potassium, 1,384 mg calcium, 3,127 mg sodium

DAY 2		SERVINGS PROVIDED							
FOOD	AMOUNT	Grains	Vegetables	Fruits	Dairy foods	Meat, poultry, & fish	Nuts, seeds, & dry beans	Fats & oils	Sweets
BREAKFAST									
prune juice	¾ cup			1					
oatmeal, cooked	½ cup	1							
whole wheat bread	1 slice	1							
soft margarine	1 tsp							1	
fat-free milk	1 cup				1				
banana	1 medium			1					
LUNCH									
BBQ beef sandwich									
lean beef	2 oz					¾			
BBQ sauce	1 tbsp								
roll	1 large	1½							
boiled potatoes	1 cup		2						
cheddar cheese, natural	1½ oz				1				
salad:									
leaf lettuce	2 leaves		½						
tomato	2 slices (¼" thick)		½						
green pepper	2 strips		½						
salad dressing, low-fat	2 tsp							⅓	
cranberry juice	1 cup			1½					
DINNER									
trout or other fish, baked									
in lemon juice	3 oz					1			
brown rice, cooked	½ cup	1							
three-bean salad:									
kidney beans	½ cup						1		
green beans	½ cup		1						
yellow beans	¼ cup		½						
Italian dressing, low-fat	4 tsp							⅔	
corn muffin	1 medium	1							
soft margarine	1 tsp							1	
spinach, cooked	½ cup		1						
SNACKS									
orange	1 medium			1					
dried fruit mixture	¼ cup (1 oz)			1					
TOTALS		**5 ½**	**6**	**5½**	**2**	**1¾**	**1**	**3**	**0**

PER DAY: 2,005 calories, 50 g total fat, 17 g saturated fat, 180 mg cholesterol, 456 mg magnesium, 4,404 mg potassium, 1,076 mg calcium, 2,579 mg sodium

DAY 3		SERVINGS PROVIDED							
FOOD	AMOUNT	Grains	Vegetables	Fruits	Dairy foods	Meat, poultry, & fish	Nuts, seeds, & dry beans	Fats & oils	Sweets
BREAKFAST									
orange juice	1 cup			1½					
cornflakes	¾ cup	1							
whole wheat bread	1 slice	1							
soft margarine	1 tsp							1	
fat-free milk	1 cup				1				
LUNCH									
sandwich:									
ham, lean, low-sodium	2 oz					¾			
cheese, reduced-fat	2 slices (1½ oz)				1				
whole wheat bread	2 slices	2							
leaf lettuce	2 leaves		½						
tomato	2 slices (¼" thick)		½						
mustard	1 tsp								
apple	1 medium			1					
DINNER									
chicken and Spanish rice	1½ cups	2	1			1			
green peas	½ cup		1						
corn muffin	1 medium	1							
melon balls	1 cup			2					
fat-free milk	1 cup				1				
SNACKS									
apricots, dried	⅓ cup (1½ oz)			1½					
almonds, unsalted	⅓ cup (1½ oz)						1		
orange	1 large			1½					
TOTALS		7	3	7½	3	1¾	1	1½	0

PER DAY: 1,987 calories, 53 g total fat, 13 g saturated fat, 153 mg cholesterol, 469 mg magnesium, 4,857 mg potassium, 1,372 mg calcium, 2,921 mg sodium

DAY 4		SERVINGS PROVIDED							
FOOD	AMOUNT	Grains	Vegetables	Fruits	Dairy foods	Meat, poultry, & fish	Nuts, seeds, & dry beans	Fats & oils	Sweets
BREAKFAST									
orange juice	1 cup			1½					
English muffin	1 whole	2							
marmalade	2 tsp								⅔
soft margarine	1 tsp							1	
fat-free milk	1 cup				1				
LUNCH									
sandwich:									
tuna, water-packed (rinsed and drained)	¼ cup					½			
whole wheat bread	2 slices	2							
iceberg lettuce	½ cup		½						
tomato	2 slices (⅛" thick)		¼						
light mayonnaise	1 tbsp							1	
carrot and celery sticks	4 sticks each		¼						
broccoli	⅔ cup		1½						
cheddar cheese, reduced-fat	1 oz				¾				
cranberry juice cocktail	½ cup			¾					
DINNER									
chicken breast, no skin	3 oz					1			
brown rice, cooked	1 cup	2							
stewed tomatoes	½ cup		1						
lima beans, cooked	½ cup		1						
spinach, cooked	⅓ cup		¾						
dinner roll	1 medium	1							
soft margarine	1 tsp							1	
fat-free milk	1 cup				1				
SNACKS									
mixed nuts, unsalted	¼ cup (1 oz)						¾		
apricots, dried	⅓ cup (1½ oz)			1½					
pretzels	¾ cup (1 oz)	1							
orange	1 medium			1					
TOTALS		**8**	**5¼**	**4¾**	**2¾**	**1½**	**¾**	**3**	**⅔**

PER DAY: 2,007 calories, 47 g total fat, 11 g saturated fat, 108 mg cholesterol, 506 mg magnesium, 4,243 mg potassium, 1,391 mg calcium, 2,074 mg sodium

DAY 5		SERVINGS PROVIDED							
Food	**Amount**	**Grains**	**Vegetables**	**Fruits**	**Dairy foods**	**Meat, poultry, & fish**	**Nuts, seeds, & dry beans**	**Fats & oils**	**Sweets**
BREAKFAST									
orange juice	1 cup			1½					
yogurt, fat-free	1 cup				1				
fruit granola bars, low-fat	2	2							
fat-free milk	1 cup				1				
banana	1 small			½					
LUNCH									
turkey sandwich:									
turkey breast	3 oz					1			
leaf lettuce	1 leaf		¼						
tomato	2 slices (¼" thick)		½						
light mayonnaise	1 tbsp							1	
whole wheat bread	2 slices	2							
carrots	7 sticks		¼						
orange, fresh	1 medium			1					
DINNER									
spicy baked fish	3 oz					1		¾	
brown rice, cooked	1 cup	2							
spinach, cooked	1 cup		2						
zucchini, cooked	½ cup		1						
dinner roll	1 medium	1							
soft margarine	2 tsp							2	
fat-free milk	½ cup				1				
melon balls	1 cup			2					
SNACKS									
peanuts, unsalted	¼ cup (1 oz)						¾		
apricots, dried	⅓ cup (1½ oz)			1½					
TOTALS		**7**	**4**	**6½**	**2½**	**2**	**¾**	**3¾**	**0**

PER DAY: 2,028 calories, 51 g total fat, 9 g saturated fat, 115 mg cholesterol, 575 mg magnesium, 5,265 mg potassium, 1,364 mg calcium, 2,411 mg sodium

DAY 6

FOOD	AMOUNT	Grains	Vegetables	Fruits	Dairy foods	Meat, poultry, & fish	Nuts, seeds, & dry beans	Fats & oils	Sweets
BREAKFAST									
orange juice	1 cup			1½					
bran flakes cereal	⅔ cup	1							
whole wheat bread	1 slice	1							
soft margarine	1 tsp							1	
fat-free milk	1 cup				1				
banana	1 small			½					
LUNCH									
chicken salad sandwich:									
chicken salad	¾ cup					1		2	
tomato	2 slices (¼" thick)		½						
whole wheat pita bread	1 small	1							
apple	1 medium			1					
DINNER									
roast beef, lean	3 oz					1			
dinner roll	1 large	1½							
baked potato	1 medium		2						
soft margarine	1 tsp							1	
green beans, cooked	¾ cup		1½						
frozen peaches	½ cup			1					
fat-free milk	1 cup				1				
SNACKS									
almonds, unsalted	⅓ cup (1½ oz)						1		
yogurt, low-fat	1 cup (1½ oz)				1				
orange juice	½ cup			¾					
TOTALS		4½	4	4¾	3	2	1	4	0

PER DAY: 2,072 calories, 55 g total fat, 12 g saturated fat, 161 mg cholesterol, 508 mg magnesium, 4,540 mg potassium, 1,320 mg calcium, 1,602 mg sodium

DAY 7

FOOD	AMOUNT	Grains	Vegetables	Fruits	Dairy foods	Meat, poultry, & fish	Nuts, seeds, & dry beans	Fats & oils	Sweets
BREAKFAST									
grape juice	1 cup			1½					
bran flakes cereal	¾ cup	1							
banana	1 medium			1					
whole wheat bread	1 slice	1							
soft margarine	1 tsp							1	
fat-free milk	1 cup				1				
LUNCH									
tuna salad sandwich:									
tuna	½ cup					1			
light mayonnaise	2 tsp							⅔	
iceberg lettuce, shredded	¾ cup		¾						
whole wheat bread	2 slices	2							
apricot nectar	¾ cup			1					
apple	1 medium			1					
DINNER									
zucchini lasagna	⅙ recipe	3	1		1				
spinach salad:									
spinach, raw	1¼ cups		1¼						
tomato	2 slices (½" thick)		1						
Parmesan cheese, grated	4 tsp				¼				
oil and vinegar									
salad dressing:									
vegetable oil	2 tsp							2	
vinegar	1 tsp								
dinner roll	1 medium	1							
soft margarine	1 tsp							1	
SNACKS									
almonds, unsalted	2 tbsp (¾ oz)						½		
raisins	⅓ cup			1½					
yogurt, fat-free	1 cup				1				
TOTALS		8	4	6	3¼	1	½	4⅔	0

PER DAY: 1,976 calories, 47 g total fat, 10 g saturated fat, 52 mg cholesterol, 506 mg magnesium, 4,290 mg potassium, 1,248 mg calcium, 1,911 mg sodium

A Comparison of Saturated Fat, Total Fat, Cholesterol, Calories, and Sodium

This table gives the saturated fat, total fat, cholesterol, calories, and sodium for some basic foods. Remember, there are 9 calories in each gram of fat. The foods within each group are ranked from low to high in saturated fat. Choose most often the foods from the top part of each group; they are lower in saturated fat and cholesterol. The examples are meant to show the difference in fat and cholesterol in select foods.

Product	Saturated Fat (grams)	Cholesterol (milligrams)	Total Fat (grams)	Total Calories	Sodium (milligrams)
MEAT, POULTRY, FISH, AND SHELLFISH (3 OZ., COOKED)					
Beef (Fat trimmed to ⅛ in unless otherwise noted)					
Liver, beef, braised*	2	331	4	137	60
Eye of round, roasted	3	60	8	171	52
Top round, broiled	3	73	8	185	51
Top sirloin, broiled	5	77	13	204	52
Ground, extra lean, broiled medium	6	71	14	217	59
Ground, lean, broiled medium	7	74	16	231	65
Salami, cooked	7	51	17	216	984
(3 oz is about 4 slices, 4 in around, ⅛ in thick)					
Chuck, arm pot roast, braised	8	86	19	277	52
Short loin, T-bone steak, broiled (¼ in trim)	9	70	18	253	52
Chuck, blade roast, braised	9	88	23	308	56
*Liver and most organ meats are low in fat but high in cholesterol					
Lamb (Fat trimmed to ⅛ in)					
Leg, whole, roasted	5	79	12	207	58
Loin, broiled	7	81	16	229	71
Shoulder, arm, braised	8	103	19	289	62
Pork (fresh unless noted otherwise) (Fat trimmed to 1/4 in)					
Cured, ham steak, boneless, extra lean, cooked, served cold	1	39	4	105	1,080
Loin, tenderloin, roasted	2	67	5	147	47
Leg (ham), rump half, roasted	5	81	12	214	52
Cured, shoulder, arm picnic, roasted	7	49	18	238	912
Ground pork, cooked	7	80	18	252	62
Chicken					
Chicken, light meat without skin, roasted	1	64	4	130	43
Breast, without skin (3 oz is about ½ breast)	1	72	3	140	63
Chicken roll, light meat, about 2 slices or 2 oz	1	27	4	87	321
Drumstick, without skin (3 oz is about 2 drumsticks)	2	79	5	146	81
Breast, with skin (3 oz is about ½)	2	71	7	168	60
Wing, without skin (3 oz is about 4 wings)	2	72	7	173	78
Chicken, dark meat without skin, roasted	3	63	7	152	81
Drumstick, with skin (3 oz is about 1½)	3	77	10	184	77

Product	Saturated Fat (grams)	Cholesterol (milligrams)	Total Fat (grams)	Total Calories	Sodium (milligrams)
Thigh, without skin (3 oz is about 1½ thighs)	3	81	9	178	75
Chicken hot dog, 1	3	55	11	142	754
Thigh, with skin (3 oz is about 1½)	4	79	13	210	71
Wing, with skin (3 oz is about 2½)	5	71	17	247	70
Turkey					
Breast, without skin	<1	71	<1	115	44
Breast, with skin	<1	77	3	130	45
Wing, without skin	1	87	3	139	66
Leg, without skin	1	101	3	135	69
Turkey roll, light meat, about 2 slices or 2 oz	1	23	4	81	269
Leg, with skin	1	60	5	145	68
Wing, with skin	2	98	8	176	62
Ground turkey, meat and skin, cooked	3	87	11	200	90
Turkey bologna, about 2 slices or 2 oz	n/a	54	8	110	483
Turkey hot dog, 1	n/a	59	10	125	785
Fish (baked, broiled, or microwaved)					
Haddock	<1	63	<1	95	74
Halibut	<1	35	3	119	59
Bluefin tuna, fresh	1	42	5	157	43
Sockeye salmon	2	74	9	183	56
Shellfish (steamed, poached, or boiled)					
Northern lobster	<1	61	<1	83	323
Clams	<1	57	2	126	95
Clams, canned, drained solids	<1	57	2	126	95
Shrimp	<1	167	1	85	192
Oyster	1	89	4	116	359
DAIRY FOODS					
Milk (1 cup)					
Skim milk	<1	4	<1	86	126
Buttermilk	1	9	2	99	257
Low-fat milk, 1% fat	2	10	3	102	123
Reduced-fat milk, 2% fat	3	18	5	121	122
Whole milk, 3.3% fat	5	33	8	150	120

Product	Saturated Fat (grams)	Cholesterol (milligrams)	Total Fat (grams)	Total Calories	Sodium (milligrams)
Yogurt (1 cup)					
Plain yogurt, nonfat	<1	4	<1	127	174
Plain yogurt, low-fat	2	14	4	144	160
Plain yogurt, whole milk	5	29	7	139	105
Soft cheeses (1 oz)					
Pot cheese or uncreamed dry curd cottage cheese, ⅓ cup	<1	3	<1	41	189
Cottage cheese, low-fat (1%), ½ cup	<1	5	1	82	459
Ricotta, part-skim, ¼ cup	3	19	5	86	78
Cottage cheese, creamed, ½ cup	3	17	5	117	457
Ricotta, whole milk, ¼ cup	5	32	8	108	52
Hard cheeses (1 oz)					
Fat-free, low-cholesterol imitation cheese	<1	1	<1	41	439
Swiss cheese, reduced fat	3	9	4	70	35
Reduced-fat and low-sodium cheese— American, cheddar, Colby, Monterey Jack, Muenster, or provolone**	3	18	4	71	88
Mozzarella, part-skim	3	16	5	72	132
Reduced-fat cheese—American, cheddar, Colby, Monterey Jack, Muenster, provolone, or string cheese**	3	15	5	79	150
Mozzarella	4	22	6	80	106
Swiss	5	26	8	107	74
American processed cheese, pasteurized	6	27	9	106	406
Cheddar	6	30	9	114	176

**The nutrient values shown for these cheeses are averages of the different types and brands.

Product	Saturated Fat (grams)	Cholesterol (milligrams)	Total Fat (grams)	Total Calories	Sodium (milligrams)
Eggs					
Egg white (1)	0	0	0	17	55
Egg yolk (1)	2	213	5	59	7
Nuts and Seeds (1 ounce—about ¼ cup—unless noted otherwise)					
(Note: All nuts and seeds are unsalted)					
Almonds	1	0	15	167	3
Sunflower seed kernels, roasted	2	0	14	165	1

Product	Saturated Fat (grams)	Cholesterol (milligrams)	Total Fat (grams)	Total Calories	Sodium (milligrams)
Pecans	2	0	19	190	0
English walnuts	2	0	17	182	3
Pistachio nuts	2	0	14	164	2
Peanuts	2	0	14	159	5
Peanut butter, smooth, made with added salt, 2 tbsp	3	0	16	190	149
Brazil nuts	5	0	19	186	0

BREADS, CEREALS, PASTA, RICE, AND DRY PEAS AND BEANS

Breads

Product	Saturated Fat (grams)	Cholesterol (milligrams)	Total Fat (grams)	Total Calories	Sodium (milligrams)
Corn tortilla, 1 (6–7 in diameter)	<1	0	<1	56	40
English muffin, 1 whole	<1	0	1	134	265
Bagel, plain, 1 (3½ in diameter)	<1	0	1	195	379
Whole wheat bread, 1 slice	<1	0	1	70	149
Hamburger or hot dog bun, plain, 1	<1	0	2	123	241
Croissant, butter, 1 medium (4½ x 4 x 1¾ in)	7	0	12	232	424

Cereals

Product	Saturated Fat (grams)	Cholesterol (milligrams)	Total Fat (grams)	Total Calories	Sodium (milligrams)
Oatmeal, instant, 1 packet (¾ cup)	<1	0	2	108	180
Oatmeal, quick, cooked without salt, 1 cup	<1	0	2	145	1
Corn flakes, 1 cup	n/a	0	<1	98	240
Granola, ½ cup	3	0	17	298	6

Pasta (1 cup cooked, without salt)

Product	Saturated Fat (grams)	Cholesterol (milligrams)	Total Fat (grams)	Total Calories	Sodium (milligrams)
Spaghetti or macaroni	<1	0	1	197	1
Egg noodles	<1	53	2	212	11

Grains (1 cup cooked, without salt)

Product	Saturated Fat (grams)	Cholesterol (milligrams)	Total Fat (grams)	Total Calories	Sodium (milligrams)
White rice	<1	0	<1	205	1
Brown rice	<1	0	2	216	9

Dry and Canned Peas and Beans (½ cup cooked)

Product	Saturated Fat (grams)	Cholesterol (milligrams)	Total Fat (grams)	Total Calories	Sodium (milligrams)
Kidney beans, canned, solids, and liquid	<1	0	1	104	445***
Kidney beans, dry, cooked without salt	<1	0	<1	112	2

Product	Saturated Fat (grams)	Cholesterol (milligrams)	Total Fat (grams)	Total Calories	Sodium (milligrams)
Garbanzo beans/chickpeas, canned, solids and liquid	<1	0	<1	143	359***
Black-eyed peas, canned, solids and liquid	<1	0	<1	92	359***

***Rinsing canned beans and peas with water
will reduce the sodium content.

FRUITS AND VEGETABLES

Fruits, raw

Product	Saturated Fat (grams)	Cholesterol (milligrams)	Total Fat (grams)	Total Calories	Sodium (milligrams)
Peach, 1	<1	0	<1	37	0
Orange, 1	<1	0	<1	62	0
Apple, 1	<1	0	<1	81	1
Banana, 1	<1	0	<1	105	1
Avocado, ⅙ (or 2 tbsp)	<1	0	5	54	4

Vegetables, cooked (½ cup)

Product	Saturated Fat (grams)	Cholesterol (milligrams)	Total Fat (grams)	Total Calories	Sodium (milligrams)
Potato	<1	0	<1	68	3
Corn	<1	0	1	89	14
Carrot	<1	0	<1	35	52
Broccoli	<1	0	<1	23	8

SWEETS

Product	Saturated Fat (grams)	Cholesterol (milligrams)	Total Fat (grams)	Total Calories	Sodium (milligrams)
Hard candy (1 oz)	0	0	0	106	11
Angel food cake, purchased, ½₂ of 9-in cake	0	0	<1	73	212
Ginger snap, 1 (about ¼ oz)	<1	0	<1	29	46
Frozen yogurt, fruit or vanilla, nonfat, ½ cup	<1	2	<1	82	39
Vanilla wafer, 1	<1	2	<1	18	12
Fig bar, 1 (about ½ oz)	<1	0	1	56	56
Pretzels, salted (1 ounce, about 5 twists, 3¼ x 2¼ x ¼ in)	<1	0	1	108	486
Popcorn, air-popped without salt (1 oz is about 3½ cups)	<1	0	1	108	1
Chocolate chip cookie, 1 (2¼ in diameter)	<1	0	2	48	32
Sherbet, orange, ½ cup	1	5	2	132	44
Ice milk, vanilla, hard, 1/2 cup	2	9	3	92	56
Potato chips, 1 oz	3	0	10	152	168
Pound cake, purchased, ¹⁄₁₀ of 10.75-oz cake	3	66	6	117	119
Ice cream, vanilla, regular, ½ cup	5	29	7	132	53

Product	Saturated Fat (grams)	Cholesterol (milligrams)	Total Fat (grams)	Total Calories	Sodium (milligrams)
FAST FOODS					
Tossed salad, no dressing, 1½ cups	0	0	<1	32	53
Grilled chicken sandwich	1	60	7	288	758
Cheese pizza, ⅛ of 12-in pizza	2	9	3	140	336
Roast beef sandwich, plain	4	52	14	346	792
French fries, regular order	4	0	12	235	124
Hamburger, plain	4	36	12	275	387
Hot dog	5	44	15	242	671
Fish sandwich with tartar sauce	5	55	23	431	615
Chicken, breaded and fried, boneless pieces, 6	6	62	18	290	542
Cheeseburger, plain, single patty	7	50	15	320	500
Chicken fillet sandwich, plain	9	60	30	515	957
Egg and bacon biscuit, 1	10	353	31	457	999
Cheeseburger, large, double patty with condiments	18	141	44	706	1,149

Product	Saturated Fat (grams)	Cholesterol (milligrams)	Polyunsaturated Fat (grams)	Monounsaturated Fat (grams)
FATS AND OILS (1 TBSP)				
Margarine, diet	1	0	2	3
Canola (rapeseed) oil	1	0	4	9
Safflower oil	1	0	11	2
Corn oil	2	0	8	4
Olive oil	2	0	1	10
Margarine, soft, tub	2	0	5	4
Margarine, liquid, bottled	2	0	5	4
Margarine, stick	2	0	4	5
Lard	5	12	2	6
Butter	7	28	<1	3

in = inches　　< = less than
oz = ounces　　n/a = not available　　tbsp = tablespoon

Sources:

Composition of Foods—Raw-Processed-Prepared, Agriculture Handbook 8. Series and Supplements, United States Department of Agriculture, Human Nutrition Information Service.

New Beef and Lamb Nutrient Data for Cuts Trimmed to 1/8 in External Fat, United States Department of Agriculture, Human Nutrition Information Service, unpublished data, 1994.

Minnesota Nutrition Data System (NDS) software, developed by the Nutrition Coordinating Center, University of Minnesota, Minneapolis, MN. Food Database version 5A, Nutrient Database version 20.

A Walking Program to Reduce Blood Pressure

A Sample Walking Program to Reduce Blood Pressure

	WARM-UP	TARGET ZONE EXERCISING*	COOL-DOWN TIME	TOTAL
WEEK 1				
Session A	Walk Normally 5 min.	Then walk briskly 5 min.	Then walk normally 5 min.	15 min.
Session B	Repeat above pattern			
Session C	Repeat above pattern			

Continue with at least three exercise sessions during each week of the program. If you find a particular week's pattern tiring, repeat it before going on to the next pattern. You do not have to complete the walking program in 12 weeks.

WEEK 2	Walk normally 5 min.	Walk briskly 7 min.	Walk normally 5 min.	17 min.
WEEK 3	Walk normally 5 min.	Walk briskly 9 min.	Walk normally 5 min.	19 min.
WEEK 4	Walk normally 5 min.	Walk briskly 11 min.	Walk normally 5 min.	21 min.
WEEK 5	Walk normally 5 min.	Walk briskly 13 min.	Walk normally 5 min.	23 min.
WEEK 6	Walk normally 5 min.	Walk briskly 15 min.	Walk normally 5 min.	25 min.
WEEK 7	Walk normally 5 min.	Walk briskly 18 min.	Walk normally 5 min.	28 min.
WEEK 8	Walk normally 5 min.	Walk briskly 20 min.	Walk normally 5 min.	30 min.
WEEK 9	Walk normally 5 min.	Walk briskly 23 min.	Walk normally 5 min.	33 min.
WEEK 10	Walk normally 5 min.	Walk briskly 26 min.	Walk normally 5 min.	36 min.
WEEK 11	Walk normally 5 min.	Walk briskly 28 min.	Walk normally 5 min.	38 min.
WEEK 12	Walk normally 5 min.	Walk briskly 30 min.	Walk normally 5 min.	40 min.

WEEK 13 ON: Check your pulse periodically to see if you are exercising within your target zone. As you get more in shape, try exercising within the upper range of your target zone. Gradually increase your brisk walking time to 30 to 60 minutes, three or four times a week. Remember that your goal is to get the benefits you are seeking and enjoy your activity.

Here's how to check if you are within your target heart rate zone:

1. Right after you stop exercising, take your pulse: Place the tips of your first two fingers lightly over one of the blood vessels on your neck, just to the left or right of your Adam's apple. Or try the pulse spot inside your wrist just below the base of your thumb.

2. Count your pulse for 10 seconds and multiply the number by 6.

3. Compare the number to the right grouping opposite: Look for the age grouping that is closest to your age and read the line across. For example, if you are 43, the closest age on the chart is 45; the target zone is 88–131 beats per minute.

AGE	TARGET HR ZONE
20 years	100–150 beats per minute
25 years	98–146 beats per minute
30 years	95–142 beats per minute
35 years	93–138 beats per minute
40 years	90–135 beats per minute
45 years	88–131 beats per minute
50 years	85–127 beats per minute
55 years	83–123 beats per minute
60 years	80–120 beats per minute
65 years	78–116 beats per minute
70 years	75–113 beats per minute

Source: Exercise and Your Heart, *National Heart, Lung, and Blood Institute and the American Heart Association, NIH Publication No. 93-1677.*

GLOSSARY

ACE (angiotensin converting enzyme) inhibitors: These drugs inhibit formation of the hormones that cause blood vessels to narrow, thus lowering blood pressure.

Alpha-beta-blocker: This medicine relaxes blood vessels and slows the heartbeat, thus reducing the blood flow to the blood vessels.

Aneurysm: A small, blisterlike out-pouching of blood vessel walls. An aneurysm can rupture, causing bleeding.

Aorta: The largest artery in the body. It conducts blood away from the heart, then branches into many smaller arteries that take the blood to the rest of the body. The diameter of the aorta enlarges with age and its walls become stiffer.

Arteries: Blood vessels that carry blood away from the heart to all parts of the body. Some enlarge with age and some become thicker and stiffer.

Atherosclerosis: A condition of the arteries in which deposits of fatty substances, cells from the artery walls, and other substances adhere to the interior artery walls, rendering them thick and irregular. This narrows the arteries. Also known as "hardening of the arteries."

Autonomic nervous system: The part of the nervous system that controls involuntary muscles such as the heart. Biofeedback has been used to affect the autonomic nervous system.

Beta-blocker: A drug that slows the heartbeat by blocking nerve impulses to the heart and blood vessels. A beta-blocker can lessen the burden on the heart.

Blood pressure (BP): Pressure of the blood against artery walls. It is recorded and monitored as two numbers: systolic before or over diastolic. The systolic pressure is the maximum pressure in the artery produced as the heart contracts and blood begins to flow. Diastolic pressure is the minimum pressure that remains within the artery when the heart is at rest.

Calcium channel blockers: These medicines prevent calcium from entering the muscle cells of the heart and blood vessels. Calcium channel blockers relax the blood vessels and decrease blood pressure.

Calories: Units of measurement that represent the amount of energy the body is able to get from foods. Different nutrients in foods provide different calorie counts. Carbohydrates and protein produce about 4 calories per gram, while fat (both saturated and unsaturated) yields about 9 calories per gram.

Capillaries: The smallest blood vessels.

Carbohydrate: One of the nutrients that supply calories to the body. Starch and fiber are complex carbohydrates. Fiber is an especially important part of the diet.

Cardiovascular: A term used to describe the heart and the blood vessels. The cardiovascular system transports oxygen and nutrients to the tissues and removes waste.

Cholesterol: A waxy substance produced by the body and taken in with food. The body makes enough cholesterol to meet its needs, such as making hormones, vitamin D, and bile acid. Cholesterol is present in all parts of the body, including the nervous system, muscle, skin, liver, intestines, and heart. When too much cholesterol circulates in the blood, one's risk of developing atherosclerosis, or "hardening of the arteries," is increased.

Diabetes mellitus: A chronic disease that may be caused by too little insulin being produced by the pancreas or the body's resistance to insulin.

Diastole: The period during a heartbeat when the chambers are filling with blood and the heart muscle is relaxed.

Diuretic: Sometimes called "water pills." A diuretic can flush excess water and sodium from the body by increasing urination. This reduces the amount of fluid in the blood and flushes sodium from the blood vessels so that they open wider, increasing blood flow and reducing blood pressure.

DNA (deoxyribonucleic acid): A large chain of molecules in the nucleus of each cell that carries the genetic information necessary for all the body's cellular functions, include the building of proteins.

EDR: The electrodermal response feedback instrument that measures skin conductivity from the fingers and palms.

ESRD: End-stage renal disease. It occurs when kidneys are destroyed by infection or toxins.

Estrogen replacement therapy (ERT): Treatment with the hormone estrogen, which has many effects, including lowering cholesterol, especially LDL.

Fat: One of the nutrients that supply calories to the body. The body needs only small amounts of fat. Foods contain different types of fat, which have different effects on blood cholesterol levels.

Fiber: Sometimes dietary fiber is called roughage. It is a part of food that cannot be digested (absorbed) by the body. It is essential for the elimination of body waste. Fiber is found in fruits, grains, and raw vegetables.

Generic drug: A medicine that has the same active ingredient as a trade-marked, brand-named version.

Heart failure: A condition in which the heart is unable to pump the amount of blood needed by the body.

High blood pressure: A persistent elevation of blood pressure above the normal range (above 140/90). Blood pressure often increases within the normal range with age. High blood pressure increases the risk of heart disease, stroke, kidney disease, and other health problems.

High-density lipoproteins (HDLs): Lipoproteins that have more protein than fat.

Hydrogenated fat: A fat that has been chemically altered by the addition of hydrogen atoms. Margarine is a hydrogenated fat. Hydrogenated fat is solid at room temperature.

Hypertension: The medical term for high blood pressure.

Hypotension: Blood pressure below normal. It can occur in shock or in some infections or diseases.

Lifestyle: An individual's way of life. This includes diet, the amount and type of physical activity in daily life, and personal habits such as sleeping, smoking, and drinking of alcoholic beverages.

Lipoprotein: A chemical compound made of fat and protein. Cholesterol and triglyceride are examples of a lipoprotein. The major lipoproteins are very low density lipoprotein (VLDL), low-density lipoprotein (LDL), and high-density lipoprotein (HDL). Each type of lipoprotein serves a different purpose and is broken down and used by the body in a slightly different way.

Milligram (mg): A unit of weight equal to one thousandth of a gram.

Milligrams/deciliter (mg/dl): The measure used to express the concentration of a chemical in the blood.

mm Hg: Abbreviation for millimeters of mercury. It is used to express measures of blood pressure. It refers to the height to which the pressure of blood against the blood vessels can push a column of mercury.

OTC: Over the counter; refers to medications that can be bought without a doctor's prescription.

PMR: Progressive muscle relaxation.

Potassium: A mineral in the body's cells necessary for maintaining fluid balance. Good sources of potassium are bananas and orange juice. Some salt substitutes contain potassium.

Risk factor: A habit, trait, or condition that is associated with an increased chance for developing a disease.

Salt: Sodium chloride is common table salt.

Saturated fat: A type of fat that raises blood cholesterol. Saturated fat is found in animal products (the white fat in raw meat), dairy products (butter, cheese, and cream), and some vegetable oils (coconut oil and palm oil). Saturated fat is solid at room temperature.

Sodium: A mineral that can contribute to high blood pressure. It is found in baking soda, some antacids, and the flavoring agent MSG (monosodium glutamate), among other items. Sodium keeps the body chemistry balanced.

Sphygmomanometer: A device used to measure blood pressure.

Stroke: A sudden loss of function in part of the brain because of loss of blood flow. Stroke may be caused by a clot (thrombosis) or rupture (hemorrhage) of a blood vessel to the brain.

Stroke volume: The amount of blood pumped with each heartbeat.

Systole: The short time during a heartbeat when the heart muscle contracts and blood is pumped into the blood vessels.

TIA: Transient ischemic attack is a disturbance in brain function resulting from a temporary deficiency in the brain's blood supply.

Triglycerides: A type of fat carried in the bloodstream. Blood triglyceride levels tend to be elevated in people who have high cholesterol levels, diabetes, or chronic kidney disease, or who are obese.

Vascular: Designates the condition of having vessels or ducts that conduct fluids, such as blood in animals or water in plants.

ADDITIONAL RESOURCES

Below is a list of organizations and resources for more information about high blood pressure. Some groups offer printed materials, others have Internet Web sites, many will provide videos. Most of the material is free, although some materials are supplied at cost, or at a minimal cost.

American Diabetes Association
1660 Duke Street
Alexandria, VA 22314
(800) 232-3472
Web site: www.diabetes.org

American Heart Association
7272 Greenville Avenue
Dallas, TX 75231-4596
(800) 242-8721
Web site: www.amhrt.org

American Society of Hypertension
515 Madison Avenue, Suite 1212
New York, NY 10022
Web site: www.ash-us.org

Mayo Clinic Health Oasis
Web site: www.mayohealth.org

National Heart, Lung, and Blood
  Institute
P.O. Box 30105
Bethesda, MD 20824-0105
Recorded information (800)
  575-9355
Web site: www.nhbi-nih.gov

National Hypertension Association
324 East 30th Street
New York, NY 10016
(212) 889-3557

National Institute of Diabetes and
  Digestive and Kidney Diseases
Office of Communications
NIDDK Information Center
P.O. Box 30105
Bethesda, MD 20824-0105
(301) 496-3583
Web site: www.niddk.nih.gov

National Kidney Foundation
30 East 33rd Street
New York, NY 10016
(800) 622-9010
Web site: www.kidney.org

National Stroke Association
96 Inverness Drive East, Suite 1
Englewood, CO 80112-5112
(800) 787-6537
Web site: www.stroke.org

Index

chicken (*cont.*)
tips about, 292
Tuscany, 297–98
see also poultry
children:
BP of, 18, 32
diet and, 105
heart disease and, 145, 148
hunger and, 90
obesity and, 81, 84, 130
sodas consumed by, 131
chili sauce, 66
chiropractic science, 234
chocolate, 311
cholesterol, 20, 29, 43, 96, 116–28, 177,
184, 260–61, 277, 325–31
alcohol and, 173–74
alternative therapies and, 233
antihypertensive drugs and, 260–61,
264–65
arteries and, 116–18, 120–21
atherosclerosis and, 24, 116–17, 122
cooking and, 308
cultures with low, 121
definition of, 117
diet and, 29, 101–2, 107–8, 111, 115–28,
145, 147–49, 221
exercise and, 120, 236
fats and, 116–26, 147
fiber and, 127–28
heart attacks and, 145, 147–48
heart disease and, 116–17, 121–22, 144–48
impotence and, 196
and learning you have HBP, 48
obesity and, 80, 83
recipes and, 310
selecting foods with low, 121
shopping and, 306
stress and, 206
stroke and, 140
cholesterol-free labels, 107, 123
chromium, 138
clothing for walking, 250
cocaine, 27, 181
coenzyme Q10, 278
coffee, 157, 171–72, 275
cognitive coping, 169
cognitive dysfunction, 188
colas, 113
colon cancer:
minerals and, 154
obesity and, 84
comfrey, 275

complementary therapies, *see* alternative
therapies
complex carbohydrates, 127, 130
condiments, 309, 315
conditioning:
hunger and, 90
obesity and, 81
Consumer Information Center (CIC), 75
Contreras, Victor, 198
convenience, overweight caused by, 93
convenience foods, 308–9
cooking of, 309
shopping for, 308
sodium in, 315
converted rice, 100–102
cookies, 90, 105, 310
low-fat, 124
oatmeal-raisin, 304
cooking, 308–10
copper, 129
corn, 72, 118, 122
corn grits, 67
corn pudding, escalloped, 291
coronary arteries, 25, 148
coronary bypass surgery, 27
coronary heart disease (CHD), 117, 128
Cottier, Christopher, 38
counseling, 218
crash diets, 93
Crazy Horse, Chief, 171
creatinine, 43, 135
Crete, 122
cross-country skiing, 253
Cryer, Philip E., 163
crying, 209
Cushing's syndrome, 82
Cutler, Jeffrey, 62
CVD, *see* cardiovascular disease

dairy products, 211, 327–28
cholesterol and, 119, 122
cooking and, 309
DASH and, 96–97, 318–24
diet and, 109, 112
minerals and, 154–56, 160
shopping for, 305–8
sodium in, 314
substitutions and, 311
women and, 192
see also butter; cheeses; milk
dancing, 208, 245
DASH, *see* Dietary Approaches to Stop
Hypertension

About the Authors

Robert L. Rowan, M.D., has been a clinical professor at New York University School of Medicine since 1977. He is noted for his ability to draw on his years of clinical experience in guiding patients in the use of self-help management techniques that have proven successful and which can be incorporated into busy lives. Dr. Rowan has authored and coauthored many previous books, including the first edition of *Control High Blood Pressure Without Drugs*, a bestseller that remained in print for nearly two decades. Most recently, he is the coauthor of *The Woman's Pharmacy*, published in 2000.

Constance Schrader, a longtime member of the American Medical Writer's Association, has authored or coauthored a dozen books in the medical and self-help fields. She has served as a staff writer for several major magazines and has written chapters on beauty and health for celebrities. Most recently, she is the author of *1001 Things Everyone Over 55 Should Know*, published in 1999. A native New Yorker, Ms. Schrader worked as a senior editor in the Macmillan and Simon & Schuster trade divisions. Ms. Schrader now lives and works in Eureka Springs, Arkansas.